Becoming a Staff Nurse

A Guide to the Role of the Newly Registered Nurse

Becoming a Staff Nurse

A Guide to the Role of the Newly Registered Nurse

Editors: Judith Lathlean and Jessica Corner

Prentice Hall
New York   London   Toronto   Sydney   Tokyo   Singapore

First published 1991 by
Prentice Hall International (UK) Limited
Campus 400, Maylands Avenue
Hemel Hempstead Hertfordshire, HP2 7EZ
A division of
Simon & Schuster International Group

Typeset in 11/13 pt Times
by Hands Fotoset, Leicester, England

Printed in Great Britain by
Redwood Books, Trowbridge, Wiltshire

Library of Congress Cataloging-in-Publication Data

Becoming a staff nurse : a guide to the role of the newly registered
  nurse / editors, Judith Lathlean and Jessica Corner.
      p.   cm.
    Includes biographical references and index.
    ISBN 0-13-072182-4
    1. Nursing.   I. Lathlean, Judith.   II. Corner, Jessica.
    [DNLM: 1. Nursing.   2. Nursing Staff, Hospital.   WY 16 B398]
  RT41.B335   1991
  610.73'06'92–dc20
  DNLM/DLC   91-3944
  for Library of Congress   CIP

British Library Cataloguing in Publication Data

Becoming a staff nurse: A guide to the role of
the newly registered nurse.
  I. Lathlean, Judith   II. Corner, Jessica
  610.73

  ISBN 0-13-072182-4

---

3 4 5   95 94

Contents

Contributors

Editors

Judith Lathlean, BSc(Econ), MA
Independent Researcher in Nursing and Research Officer,
Department of Educational Studies, Oxford University

Jessica Corner, BSc, PhD, RGN
Senior Macmillan Lecturer and Head of Academic Nursing Unit,
Institute of Cancer Research, Royal Marsden Hospital, London

Contributors

Angela Heslop, Dip N, RCNT, RGN
Senior Nurse, Nursing Development Unit and Respiratory Health Worker,
Charing Cross Hospital, London

Richard McMahon, MA, Dip N, RGN
Senior Nurse, Care of the Elderly
Horton Hospital, Banbury

Caroline Shuldham, MSc, PGCEA, Dip N, RCNT, RNT, RGN
Director of Education,
Royal Brompton National Heart and Lung Hospitals Special Health Authority

Ingrid Stevens, RCNT, Royal Marsden Oncological Nursing Certificate, RGN
Lecturer Practitioner,
Churchill Hospital/Oxford Polytechnic

Barbara Vaughan, MSc, Dip N, RCNT, RNT, DANS, SRN
Senior Lecturer
School of Nursing Studies, University of Wales College of Medicine

Introduction

Becoming a staff nurse is one of the biggest steps that nurses take. For many the transition from being a student to a fully qualified practitioner is challenging and stressful. Yet only relatively recently have the problems and difficulties of taking on the first post following training been studied systematically with a view to seeing what might be done to improve the situation. A research study by Lathlean *et al.* (1986) evaluated three specially established schemes aimed at the professional development of newly registered nurses. The schemes were set up on the assumption that nurses do need help and support in their first staff nurse post and that this help can best be provided in a combined clinical and educational setting. But the study proved to be much more than an evaluation of strategies to develop nurses; it highlighted the inadequacy of basic training to prepare nurses for a whole range of activities including planning and assessing patient care; ward management; communication with patients, their relatives and with some groups of staff; teaching; and coping with death and dying. In addition, it identified the stress that is experienced by many nurses in coping with their new role in an environment which is constantly changing.

The insights gained from this study, and the rich case material provided by a large number of newly registered nurses, stimulated the writing of this book. The editors, together with the contributors, all of whom work with recently qualified nurses and have first hand knowledge of their needs, have attempted to address important aspects of the staff nurse role so that those embarking on it may have a better understanding of it. In doing so, they have drawn on their considerable experience as well as on relevant research and literature. The book is further intended to give practical help and information to assist not only students about to qualify and nurses when just qualified, but also those who are more senior and who want to review their roles, as well as people whose responsibility it is to support and develop them, such as sisters and educators. It is not intended as a panacea, nor should it give the message that all newly registered nurses will find themselves in the same position when taking up their first post. Indeed, Lathlean's research showed that individuals vary greatly in their needs and concerns. It might be of value for the reader to consider the extent to which the research findings highlight a familiar or unfamiliar situation to the one that they have experienced, or are about to go through.

At long last the importance of professional development for all who have completed their initial training is being recognised. Programmes and opportunities aimed at the needs of staff nurses and sisters are becoming more usual, though it will still be some time before all nurses will automatically be offered the chance to develop their skills and learning further. It is hoped that this book with its research- and experience-based information will be a useful source book of insight and ideas, either as part of a programme or plan or for the individual who is interested in being an effective staff nurse.

Nursing is in the process of considerable change and much has happened in the last few years that is altering the role and preparation of the staff nurse. Nursing practice, education and management are all in a state of flux and the possible effects of the major developments – such as the reform of initial nurse education, the plans for continuing education and the move towards primary nursing as a way of organising care – are considered. But perhaps one of the most important aspects of a nurse's role that has been stressed recently is that of accountability. The fact that each registered nurse is accountable for the care that they provide for patients, from the day that the student passes the exams for registration and chooses to practise as a nurse, is critical. This has great implications for nurses themselves and for those who manage them and assist in their education. This book touches on many areas in which new nurses can be helped, by the development of knowledge, skills and attitudes, to be more confident and able to accept their accountability.

Reference

Lathlean, J., Smith, G. and Bradley, S. (1986) *Post-Registration Development Schemes Evaluation*, Kings College, University of London.

A note on gender terminology

Within this text, in the interests of uniformity of approach, the nurse will be referred to as she, the patient as he.

1 The Role of the Staff Nurse

JUDITH LATHLEAN

Introduction

Though nurse education is in the midst of change, nurses have for many decades been prepared in an apprenticeship system; that is, 'an exclusive method of training or of preparing young persons for a craft, a skill, an employment or a profession, which involves the attachment of the trainees for an agreed period of time to a specific member of that profession'. (Singer and Macdonald 1970). While they are members of the workforce during training, student nurses, however senior, *are* different from qualified nurses. Most obviously they wear different uniforms and embellishments (belts, ribbons, and the like) to delineate their status and year of training. Also they are prevented from undertaking certain nursing tasks considered to be the province only of qualified nurses, but, perhaps most importantly, they are not deemed to be accountable professional practitioners and are viewed differently by others – nursing staff, doctors, health care workers and patients and their relatives.

On registration, they are supposed to be competent, clinically knowledge-able and skilled, able to manage the planning and implementation of the care of a group of patients, well organised and capable of taking charge of the ward, adept at answering telephone calls, even in difficult circumstances such as breaking bad news to relatives, confident in their dealings with doctors, and good teachers of, and role models for students, the ranks of whom they have only just left. The reality is – and this has been borne out by research – that many newly qualified nurses are not competent and confident in all these and other facets of their new role. This chapter seeks to explore the difficulties and challenges experienced in the move from student to staff nurse, before considering the present – and future – role of the staff nurse. Aspects of the role are examined in more detail in the subsequent chapters.

1

From student to staff nurse

Despite variation between individuals, the research by Lathlean *et al.* (1986) indicated that many nurses find the transition from being a student to a staff nurse difficult and feel unprepared for their new role. This was also shown in an earlier study by Vaughan (1980) of factors affecting the transition and reinforced by a later study by Humphries (1987). (For the synopses of these latter two pieces of research, please see Appendix 1.1)

Does basic training adequately prepare for the role?

During the exploratory work for Vaughan's research, one of the respondents said: 'We are trained to pass an exam . . ., not to run a ward, how to cope with difficult doctors and relatives and how to treat consultants', a view reflected by over a quarter of nurses in the main sample who argued that *no* area of their training had been helpful in preparing them to cope with different aspects of the staff nurse role. The researcher goes on to conclude: 'Although it may be suggested that this view is exaggerated, since the respondents must have learnt something in order to be able to practise as qualified nurses, it does indicate that there are parts of their role that have been neglected in training.' (Vaughan 1980).

Vaughan also asked for suggestions of subjects which could be included in the general training in order to prepare the student better for her new role on registration. By far the highest proportion of comments referred to 'management', including management principles and skills (such as legal knowledge and ordering), and a clearer understanding of the role of the staff nurse and others within the nursing hierarchy. Other aspects mentioned (in descending order of frequency) were: the opportunity to practise, behavioural sciences, counselling, and teaching skills.

There have been many changes in nurse training in the past ten years, as discussed in Chapter 3, and it might be thought that the situation found by Vaughan has altered quite a lot since 1980. However, Humphries (1987) more recently asked a group of newly qualified nurses the same set of questions as Vaughan and found that although the proportion of nurses who said that *no* aspect of the training had prepared them for their role was much smaller (10 per cent of all respondents), inadequate preparation was still highlighted as one of the most important reasons why difficulties were experienced in transition from student to staff nurse. Management practice again featured high on the list of requests for inclusion in basic training followed by: a deeper knowledge base; interpersonal skills; and personal supervision and support.

Better initial preparation is not of course the complete answer. Pre-registration training provides a set of principles for the new nurse, but, according to Benner (1984), until the nurse has learnt to make judgements about their relative importance, she is unable to move away from them. Newly qualified nurses are novices in this respect and need to go through many phases before becoming (if ever) 'expert practitioners' (see Chapter 2 for a more detailed description of Benner's ideas). Thus initial training should set the framework for practice as a nurse; but only through further learning and by being able to draw on a repertoire of experiences as a qualified nurse will the individual develop high-level skills and competence.

Expectations of the staff nurse role

One factor of importance in the transition from student to staff nurse is the overall expectation that students have of the role. In a study which looked at the perceptions of the staff nurse role it was found that first year students held perceptions about the staff nurse role that were very different from those of the staff nurses themselves, whereas by the second year, these perceptions were much more similar. The views of third year students concurred with those of staff nurses, except that third year students thought that the clinical aspects of the job were significantly less important than did the staff nurses (Buckenham 1988). The author concludes that this discrepancy is probably due to emphasis placed on management functions during the final year of training at the expense of the clinical function, yet many newly qualified nurses still feel most unprepared in the area of management.

This change in perception is in line with the distinction described by Davis (1975) in which new recruits to nursing (in the United States) enter with a 'lay imagery' of the role of the nurse which, through a process of socialisation, becomes an 'institutionally approved imagery' (that is, based on the school's ethos of nursing) by the completion of training. Davis (1975) argues that 'the beginning student's simplistic assumption that satisfactory nursing performance entails little more than a kind and caring attitude in league with an instrumental ability 'to do for' the patient is replaced by a perspective which views the nurse's very relationship to the patient in problematic terms'. Others describe this change as the socialisation of the lay person to a professional role (for example, Simpson et al. 1979), and it is suggested that one of the tasks of nurse educators is to prepare students for the standards of performance which are expected of them as professionals (Claus and Bailey 1977).

Clearly, many processes take place during the initial training which alter students dramatically – in terms of their knowledge, skills, attitudes and perceptions. It is known that relationships between student nurses and those responsible for influencing them during their training are of great importance. Davis (1983), in a British research study of the relationships between student nurses and their 'significant others', suggests that 'these relationships are of particular relevance to the development of the self-image, socialisation into the role of nurse and the ability to cope with various nursing related problems'. On becoming a staff nurse, it seems that whilst the majority find the role as they had expected (Vaughan 1980; Humphries 1987), there are surprises for some nurses, in fact for a third of the sample in Humphries' (1987) study. For example, whilst a few had not anticipated the increased responsibility and workload, others had imagined the responsibility and the respect to be greater than it actually was. This is clearly disappointing to some nurses; one nurse in Humphries' study commented: '[The role of staff nurse] is as I expected – but not as I would like it to be!'

How different is it from being a student?

Leaving aside the students' expectations, what are the actual differences between being a third year student and a staff nurse? Matthewson (1985) says that there is no difference in the nurses themselves; rather the difference lies in how other people see the newly qualified nurse and what expectations they have of them. But it is more than that. In her study, Vaughan (1980) asked the nurses to identify the aspects of their work that were most different now that they were qualified. Over 80 per cent of the sample said that colleagues and/or patients and relatives behaved differently now that they were qualified. Almost three-quarters noted that decision making, planning and the responsibility for others were greatly enhanced, with half feeling that administration and paper work had increased. Only 13 per cent mentioned loss of patient contact.

Humphries (1987) found overall the same response except that an even higher proportion (84 per cent) noted the increased responsibility, and slightly less (50 per cent) the altered relationships. In the case of the latter, many specifically commented that other people's expectations of them had increased and changed: the nurse was 'suddenly expected to know everything' and her 'opinions were sought and listened to'.

Difficulties and needs of newly qualified nurses

While for many nurses the transition from student to staff nurse is as expected, and for some no great difficulties are experienced, for others it is a 'shock' and brings feelings of 'dread, terror and fear' (Lathlean *et al.* 1986). Kramer (1974) describes these feelings among American nurses as 'Reality Shock' and suggests that the reason for them is the variance between the real and the ideal world. In order to cope, nurses can follow one of various options; these are discussed in Chapter 2. In the United Kingdom, most students are currently exposed to the 'reality' much earlier on, and therefore such experiences should be less prevalent and not as profound. It is interesting to consider, however, whether this situation will change with the implementation of Project 2000 programmes, when students will be supernumerary for the majority of their training and only giving 20 per cent of rostered service towards the end of the course.

Some aspects of the job are obviously more problematic than others. For example, Vaughan (1980) identified that just over half found delegation and co-ordination difficult, nearly a third had problems with staff relations; and almost a fifth, in talking to relatives. In Humphries' (1987) study, the situation seems to have improved slightly in respect of some aspects: between a fifth and a quarter of the nurses surveyed found difficulty with increased responsibility, delegation and staff relations; smaller proportions mentioned teaching and relationships with relatives. In both studies, nurses were asked why they thought these difficulties had arisen and the reasons given (in descending order of importance for each study) were: staff attitudes (lack of understanding between themselves and other members of the health care team), inadequate preparation, personal insecurity and lack of time (Vaughan 1980), and role conflict (where the workload makes combined clinical and managerial demands and the inability to complete either aspect satisfactorily), feelings of being unprepared, relation-ships with staff (including 'not being liked by other staff', being ignored by staff when in charge, being treated 'differently' and 'indifferently' by the doctors and more experienced nurses) and nurses' insecurity (Humphries 1987).

The research by Lathlean *et al.* (1986) took a different approach. Instead of asking only nurses what difficulties they were experiencing, it attempted to find out what were the needs for development and support of staff nurses, as seen by them, their tutors and managers. It identified two groups of needs: 'those containing qualities which vary according to the specific role and tasks of the nurse (called task related needs) and those in which developments are very relevant to her present role but will also continue to be relevant in all her future roles, both in nursing and outside (called developmental needs)' (Lathlean *et al.* 1986). The needs were found to vary between different individuals, so a range of areas in which any one person should develop in the first six to ten months of practice, and the possible extent of those needs were explored.

In the first group – task related needs – the following needs were found:

Management of individual patient care

Few nurses were able to articulate clearly the concepts of the nursing process; 'often no reference was made to individualised patient care or to systematic assessment, planning, implementation and evaluation. . . . Managers and/or tutors identified gaps in the newly registered nurses' practice of individual patient care management, . . . such as long term planning of a patient's care, involvement of patients in their care, and satisfactory completion of the evaluation component in care plans, although these were not mentioned by the nurses themselves.' (Lathlean *et al.* 1986).

Ward management

Almost every participant mentioned this as a need, though the term appeared to be associated with a wide range of skills and qualities. Examples of the problems encountered included: writing up doctors' rounds and passing on the appropriate information; drawing up the duty rota; knowing how to get help from outside the ward; and knowledge of district policies and procedures.

Clinical skills and knowledge

Most of the nurses felt that their training had prepared them adequately for non-specialist clinical tasks, but observations by ward sisters and tutors showed that this assumption was not always borne out in practice. Furthermore, even where the nurse was deemed to be clinically competent by such people, there were still some inadequacies, particularly the sometimes uncritical acceptance of traditional clinical procedures and, linked with this, the need for greater awareness and application of research-based knowledge.

Understanding the role

Just as the first few months of nurse training entails 'learning the role of the student nurse' (Davis 1983), so the first few months post-registration was seen to be 'learning the role of the staff nurse'. This included learning the specific knowledge and skills necessary, but, in addition, some nurses were unsure of what the role actually comprised. For some, it was the oscillations that were most confusing; 'You go from being in charge one day and back to being a student the next.' This lack of clarity of role seems to extend more generally to the role of the nurse, not just when newly registered. For example, when and under what circumstances should a nurse challenge a medical decision, clear up after doctors, make telephone calls for them and so on? Whilst the clinical grading structure for nurses has attempted to clarify in general terms the responsibilities and expectations of the nurse, there will still be enormous variations between nurses in any one grade.

Communication with patients and relatives

Two major problem areas emerged: responding to the psychological (emotional) needs of patients and coping with a dying patient and his relatives. In relation to the first area, Menzies (1960) identified the tendency for nurses to busy themselves with the technical tasks of nursing, as a protection against involvement and a 'defence against anxiety'. Responding to emotional needs makes the nurse more vulnerable and may be one of the reasons for the difficulties observed. Also the necessary skills and knowledge of how to communicate may not be sufficiently well developed at this stage, hence the avoidance of such situations or the poor handling of them. (Chapter 4 addresses many of the relevant issues here.)

Newly qualified nurses were particularly concerned with their relationships with dying patients and their relatives, especially where it was unclear how much information should be given. Nurses felt ill-prepared to inform relatives of a patient's death and did not know 'how to respond to the bereaved and distressed relatives, including the extent to which the nurse should be open about her own grief, and how to manage the feelings of inadequacy she experienced' (Lathlean *et al.* 1986). (This important area is touched upon in Chapter 4 and considered in depth in Chapter 7.)

Communication with other staff

In terms of nurses' communication with other staff, problems were identified in two main respects: the first was finding an effective way of relating to staff in order to ensure that ward work was completed, and the second, in their relationships with doctors. Many newly qualified nurses had difficulty in exerting authority, gaining respect and reprimanding staff, and they reacted by 'giving up', or being 'bossy' or 'condescending'. Although most nurses described their relationships with doctors as 'good', problems were found where there were divergences between nursing and medical opinion and where the nurse felt unjustly criticised.

Teaching and expression of ideas

The study found that most of the nurses lacked skills in certain areas of teaching, for example: finding out the learner's level of understanding and needs; clearly identifying what they were setting out to teach; and giving sufficient explanation. Guidance was also required for those responsible for continuous assessment of students including writing reports and how to give feedback. There was concern about giving formal teaching sessions on the ward; some felt the need for greater articulacy as well as help with structure and content. The concern also extended to the expression of views with colleagues in group discussions and debates.

In the second group – developmental needs – the following areas of concern were found:

Decision making and analytical thought

Many of the nurses were considered, especially by ward sisters, to be poor organisers, both of the ward and of their own work. This seemed to stem from problems with decision making, and the inability to take an overall view of a situation, assess priorities and plan ahead. This problem has been identified by Benner (1984) who argues that it is only when the 'novice' nurse moves to the stage of 'advanced beginner' that she starts to take a more global view (see Chapter 2). Some nurses showed little autonomy, in terms of their ability and willingness to make decisions without support and advice. Again, Benner (1984) suggests that novice nurses are unable to draw on past experiences in order to make decisions; they have learnt a set of principles but do not yet have the judgement required to move away from them. In addition, the nurse's capacity to organise seemed to be related to the degree of stress; the more under pressure the nurse became, the more her organisational skills 'went to pot'.

In terms of analytical thought, the problems seem to emanate from the tendency of some nurses to see things in 'black and white', though doubtless the changing nature of basic training which encourages analysis and enquiry will eventually change this. The nurses themselves were often not aware of any deficiencies, but tutors and managers identified a lack of depth of thought.

Uncritical acceptance of the work culture

There was a tendency for the nurses to accept without questioning the established work culture – the prevailing methods and attitudes – even when these were contrary to the nurse's own beliefs and view. Sometimes it was more the result of a lack of individual thought rather than an inability to challenge, but as one nurse explained 'The training seems to knock out of you any individual thought or creativity; you're there to pass your exams'. There was also the sense of getting into a routine and not being so aware of deficiencies. The person moving to a new home may have good intentions of changing this and improving that, but after a few months the urgency seems to fade and one becomes less aware of the flaking paint and the hideous wall paper. In a similar way, the new nurse may feel: 'I've been here six months and I've got into the organisation now. You get into the routine of how everybody does it and just get used to that way.'

There was also some lack of confidence in expressing criticism of the status quo, not always helped by the attitudes of some of the staff. So the nurses tended to find it more comfortable to 'fit in' and do what was expected.

Unused potential

Several nurses appeared capable of making a great contribution to patient care and to nursing as a whole, but seemed stifled, possibly by an inability to exert autonomy. In one instance, the nurse was described by her managers as 'capable of anything at the moment'. Nevertheless, even she 'had difficulty varying from routine and challenging inappropriate patient care', and finding ways of making the improvements needed on the ward.

Self-awareness and self-confidence

Achieving a balance between lack of awareness of personal capabilities and limitations and a heightened awareness of weaknesses seemed difficult for most. Thus, at one end of the scale there were nurses with insufficient sensitivities to their own shortcomings, whilst, at the other extreme, were nurses who were 'too aware' of their weaknesses and unable (or unwilling) to identify their own strengths, leading to a diminution of self-confidence.

Self-awareness and self-confidence seemed to go hand in hand – those who were most self-aware without being too negative tended to feel the most confident. However, the term 'confident' is used here to convey a 'sense of security which is *soundly-based* on the nurse's awareness of her own capabilities, values and rights' and not as sometimes used, 'to describe a characteristic more related to conformity to tradition or established expectations of the staff nurse role' (Lathlean *et al.* 1986).

Response to stress
In some nurses the response to stress sometimes had adverse consequences for patient care, for their relationships with other staff and for their own health. Reactions varied: for example, blocking out the stressful incidents and denying they had happened; being flippant and superficial; complaining unconstructively; becoming apathetic, withdrawn and even leaving the job. Some of the tutors noticed the phenomenon of 'post-registration depression' – the occurrence of disillusionment and apathy about three months after registration. (See Chapter 6 for a more detailed discussion of stress and stress management.)

Awareness of professional philosophy and current issues
Most of the nurses studied had limited awareness and understanding of current nursing philosophy. For example: they were hazy about the appropriate role of the nurse and the nurses' relationship to doctors; they were unsure of, or ambivalent towards changing concepts of managing nursing care (such as the nursing process); they appeared not to have grasped the concept of continuing education; research, budgetary issues and even accountability were of limited interest. The issues most burning to the nurses tended to be salaries and financial cutbacks: few had much knowledge of major influences affecting nursing as a whole such as the Griffiths Report (a major issue at the time) and none mentioned the impending changes in basic nurse education (now published as Project 2000 – UKCC, 1986).

Career planning
The picture was one of contrasts: the group of nurses who had no clear idea of what they would be doing beyond the next few months compared with those who were planning on embarking on a 'typical' career pathway (such as gaining experience in medicine and surgery, followed by post-registration training), often planned whilst a student, but not necessarily revised in the light of their

changing views or the needs of the service. The study concluded that newly registered nurses need the following:

- information about the possible opportunities;
- help to explore common assumptions about suitable career paths;
- assistance in viewing the context of their work more broadly;
- individual guidance from someone who knows them well enough to give them accurate feedback on their capabilities;
- guidance and support in putting their plans into action (Lathlean *et al.* 1986).

Factors facilitating the transition

Given this large number of possible areas of need for development in the newly qualified nurse what are some of the factors that assist in the transition from a student through to a senior staff nurse, and perhaps further? Vaughan (1980) asked her respondents whether any member of the ward team had affected this adjustment to the new role in a positive way, and nearly 82 per cent said yes. The most helpful person (by far) was the ward sister, followed by a state enrolled nurse, staff nurse and ward clerk. The positive help took the form of: advice and guidance (most usually); personal relationships; expression of confidence; and role modelling. When asked if they had had any other help in adjusting, just over half said yes, and included: senior nursing staff, inservice course, peer group support, medical staff and final block of training.

It is interesting to find that in Humphries' (1987) research three-quarters identified a member of the ward team who had helped them positively, and that this person was usually a staff nurse (twenty-seven responses), followed by sister (twelve responses). Most often the help took the form of support and reassurance (67 per cent of responses), though sometimes it took the form of practical help or by the person acting as a role model. Other help from outside the ward team came mainly from friends, though staff nurses and doctors received several mentions. They were described as helpful because they were: 'supportive and readily available'; 'helpful, gave advice, explained things'; 'patient and willing to listen'; or 'encouraging and praised the nurse'.

The research by Lathlean *et al.* (1986) compared developments occurring in a group of nurses who went through a professional development programme with a group who did not, and found that the extent of development was greater in all but one of the programme members than in the non-participants. This seems to indicate that the programme was beneficial for the majority in helping them through their first six to nine months post-registration. Features of the programme included: support and advice from facilitators (tutors and sisters); guided practice with feedback; and structured learning opportunities such as study days, projects, reading time, and event diaries.

The role of staff nurse

A picture of the role of the staff nurse is already beginning to emerge, but, as a prelude to the rest of the book, the main aspects of the role will be considered briefly. First, though, it is important to look at the work that has been undertaken, and views that have been expressed about the nature of the nurse's role and the proportion of time that staff nurses spend on different activities.

The nature of the role

Perhaps one of the best known and still widely accepted definitions of the role of the nurse is that of Virginia Henderson (1966):

> The unique function of the nurse is to assist the individual, sick or well, in the performance of those activities contributing to health or its recovery (or a peaceful death) that he would perform unaided if he had the strength, will or knowledge, and to do this in such a way as to help him gain independence as rapidly as possible.

But as Henderson (1979) points out, over a decade later, nursing must be seen as part of the social scene, and that of course is changing all the time, as are the economic, political, cultural and value systems of society. One of the major effects of this has been a shift away from nursing as just being about sickness (sometimes described as a 'biomedical' model) to a view that nursing 'is concerned with man as a total being at some point along a health–illness continuum' (Roy 1970). The role of the nurse then includes assessment to find out a person's position on the health–illness continuum, and intervention to help that person make suitable adaptation.

The increasing use of nursing 'models' has highlighted the changed beliefs about nursing which tend in turn to affect the role of the nurse. Pearson and Vaughan (1986) suggest that the various models seem to agree on a number of concepts about patients and nursing, and the main ones are the following:

- health;
- the holistic view of people;
- the humanistic view of people;
- the autonomy of patients and clients;
- the need to develop a productive or therapeutic relationship between those who nurse, and those who are nursed.

(For further discussion of nursing models see also Kershaw and Salvage 1986.)

The 'biomedical' model 'has led to an emphasis on the technical, medically-related aspects of the nursing role and to a resulting devaluation of acts related to how individuals are experiencing their own illnesses or disabilities, such as listening, comforting or the offering of choices' (Pearson and Vaughan 1986).

Yet this model is prevalent in nursing today; there are still many wards where the more senior nurse will perform the cure-directed acts such as giving drugs and performing dressings, the more junior nurses or students will provide physical care such as bathing because of their 'lesser' technical knowledge, and the orientation is towards physical aspects of care. In this environment, the student might feel on qualification that her role will change to that of 'curer' rather than that of physical carer that she has experienced as a student. There are clear disadvantages to this way of nursing, however. For example, it leads to patients being labelled with a diagnosis rather than being treated as whole human beings and it concentrates information and knowledge with the doctors, minimising the rights of patients and the therapeutic role of the nurse.

The concepts of holism (where individuals are considered to be different from and more than the sum of their parts), humanism (a system which recognises that man is a responsible and progressive intellectual being), autonomy of patients (acknowledging that people should have choice in their care and the right to be involved in this process), and partnership in the nurse/patient relationships (as opposed to the nurse directing practice for the client) are fulfilled in ways of organising nursing that are different from the traditional patterns. Thus forms of organisation such as team nursing and primary nursing incorporating individualised patient care, which promote these concepts, are replacing the hierarchical prescription of care based on tasks. When this happens, the role of the nurse is fundamentally altered. For example, she is far more autonomous (whereby autonomy is the freedom to make decisions within the limits of competence of the individual) and is accountable for the total care of individual patients.

Time spent on various activities

Using a different approach, some have looked at the different activities of nurses and have tried to identify the proportions of time spent on each type. For example, Moores and Moult (1979) undertook systematic activity sampling of nursing auxiliaries, students and pupils, and trained nurses (including staff nurses and sisters) and found that the more qualified the grade of nurse, the larger the proportion of time that was spent on administrative duties. They identified over 130 potential tasks performed by the grades that they studied and grouped them into six categories: basic (e.g. bathing a patient and providing a bedpan); technical (e.g. giving drugs and doing dressings); administrative (e.g. completing patient's records and drawing up a duty rota); personal; unskilled and other. The average proportion of a staff nurse's time spent on administrative tasks was 50 per cent (21 per cent for third year students); on basic nursing tasks it was 25 per cent (47 per cent for third year students); and for technical tasks it was 17 per cent (18 per cent for third year students). The amount of time spent on other activities was very small.

Both Vaughan and Humphries asked staff nurses to rate five items in terms of the amount of time that they took each day: ward administration e.g. paperwork, ordering; communication with other professionals (e.g. doctors); giving direct clinical care; supervising others giving clinical care; and teaching (nurses, patients and relatives). Vaughan (1980) found that 'significantly more people spend the greatest proportion of their time in communicating with other professionals and the least amount of their time in teaching either students, patients or relatives'. In addition, just under a half of the respondents ranked direct clinical care and one-third of the respondents ranked ward administration as the most or the second to most time consuming activity. Humphries' (1987) results were similar though there was an even greater shift towards communication and clinical care and a move away from ward administration. Communication with professionals was highlighted as most time consuming with over two-thirds of the respondents; but direct clinical care was not far behind – over half of the respondents ranked this highly. Conversely, teaching was least time consuming for over half, as was ward administration.

Although the results of the Moores and Moult study are not directly comparable with those of Vaughan and Humphries, because the groupings of activities are not the same, they do seem to indicate that there has been a tendency for management and administration to be taking up a diminishing proportion of time for an increasing number of staff nurses. The pattern of results found in the latter two studies does show the variation between staff nurse jobs, particularly in relation to the amount of time they spend on different activities. In addition, as has been discussed above, changing systems and ways of organising nursing alter the role of the staff nurse. However, there are many common elements to the job – it tends to be the emphasis upon them that varies.

The different aspects of the role

In theory it might be thought that the newly registered nurse, being the least experienced trained nurse on the ward, would be accountable for care given to a group of allocated patients, but would only gradually be eased into greater responsibility. In practice, many new nurses have wide ranging responsibilities and 'in some instances much of the work of the newly registered nurse differs little from that of the senior staff nurse or ward sister' (Lathlean et al. 1986). However, this does depend on a variety of factors, especially the staffing levels on the ward, the skill mix (the balance of trained to untrained staff and the degree of experience of the nurses), the way that the nursing is organised on the ward and the role, behaviour and attitudes of the nurse in charge. For example, where staffing levels allow, and where the sister has a policy of not allowing recently qualified nurses to be in charge without the support of a more senior nurse, the role of the more junior nurse is differentiated from that of the seniors. It remains to be seen how the role of the health care assistant (support worker) affects the differentiation of the role of the staff nurse.

Clinical grading has had an impact in this respect with its more precise delineation of responsibilities. So, for example, a newly registered nurse on a D grade is not expected to be in charge of the ward regularly, whereas a staff nurse on an E grade is expected to carry out all relevant forms of care *and* to take charge regularly in the absence of the person who has continuing responsibility.

Most newly qualified nurses have a major part to play in the *provision of clinical care,* though their role in this has been extended, expanded and changed over the years. There have been many debates over the topics of giving intravenous drugs and the extent to which patient assessment should include an element of physical assessment which verges on the diagnostic role of the doctor. Some nurses resent this and feel they are expected to be mini-doctors, or combined medics, social workers and nurses; others see it as an important and necessary move towards the recognition of nursing as a unique professional discipline. (This is exemplified by the establishment in some hospitals of nursing units, which seeks 'to promote high quality nursing and, in doing so, the development of clinical nursing as a discipline through its practice, education and research' (Pearson 1983).) In addition, with the increased emphasis on the therapeutic nature of nursing, some nurses are trying out different 'alternative' or complementary approaches to care, such as massage and aromatherapy, which require an extension of the traditional clinical skills. The role of the newly registered nurse in providing clinical care is explored further in Chapter 2.

Management and administrative activities form a significant part of the role of many new staff nurses. Many do not feel that they possess the necessary skills and knowledge for this part of their job, and even those who are relatively confident lack some abilities in areas such as planning and organising the ward work; managing their own workload and that of a team; delegation and supervision; use of resources including ordering and utilisation of supplies; understanding and budgeting; planning patient discharge; and knowledge of disciplinary and grievance procedures and health and safety at work. These and many other topics are considered in Chapter 3.

Communication between nurses, patients and their relatives, and between the nurse and other staff is an area that many new staff nurses found to be particularly difficult in Lathlean *et al.*'s (1986) research. Chapter 4 highlights some of the considerations and problems including: the factors that are important in good communication at ward level; dealing with patients and their relatives; relating to the 'difficult' or 'unpopular' patient; talking to worried or bereaved relatives; and communicating with other members of the nursing team and with doctors and the health care team.

Although many new staff nurses see *teaching* as only a small part of their role, certainly in terms of the amount of time they consider they spend on it, this is due in part to the feeling that many have that teaching is about 'imparting knowledge' to others in a fairly formal way. Teaching and learning are of course intertwined and if the nurse thinks of herself as a creator of learning opportunities, as well as a beneficiary of opportunities, this more accurately reflects the processes that occur. Chapter 5 explores the topic, indicating the nature of learning and teaching, and highlighting some opportunities for learning.

Coping with the staff nurse role

Given the increasing demands of the job of staff nurse it is hardly surprising that Lathlean's study found that 'most of the nurses . . . experienced strain during the six month period [of the research] and that many of the factors apparently affecting this were directly related to their positions as newly registered nurses' (Lathlean *et al.* 1986). The nurses who did not feel some strain tended either to have benefited from a supported induction to their new role or, alternatively, were lacking in self-awareness and relatively 'immune' to the pressures. The strain of the transition and the new role gave rise to stress in many individuals.

Lathlean *et al.* (1986) identified a number a factors which appear to give rise to stress in the new role. These include the following:

- being in charge of the ward (the responsibility, the need to establish authority, the demands and the relationships with particular groups, notably doctors);
- other aspects of the role such as contact with relatives, coping with dying patients, certain clinical tasks, and supporting and developing students;
- the lack of clarity of the role;
- the inadequacy of support and feedback;
- external factors such as standards on the ward, problems of staffing, staff relations and working conditions.

Stress and ways of responding to stress are the subject of Chapter 6. Referring to the variety of potential 'stressors', coping with death and dying was found to be one of the most problematic aspects. This is discussed at length in Chapter 7.

The way forward

The ever changing nature of nursing, and the many developments that have occurred in the past decade and are continuing to influence the nature and shape of nursing practice, education and management means that a book of this kind can become quickly out of date. However, throughout there has been an attempt to consider the range of innovations and new ways of working and suggest how these may impinge on the role of the novice staff nurse. Chapter 8 brings together some of the most important changes that have taken place as well as those which have yet to be fully implemented.

Although many newly qualified nurses have little idea of their future career beyond the next six months to a year (Lathlean *et al.* 1986), the opportunities in nursing are diverse and exciting. As a result of the new clinical grading structures and the effects of other developments, such as the realisation that clinical practice is at the heart of good nursing, it is now increasingly possible and desirable for a nurse to stay in clinical practice and receive commensurate financial rewards. Alternatively, the preference may be to focus on a type of nursing, such as intensive care or oncology or on the nursing of particular client groups or specialties such as paediatrics, care of the elderly, mental handicap, or mental illness. For others, the lure of management, education or research is great, or a move to midwifery, district nursing or health visiting is desirable. Many of these avenues require a further period of post-registration training, but even if the nurse wishes solely to practise as a staff nurse, the consolidation of the initial preparation and opportunities for professional development and continuing education are important. These are discussed in Chapter 9.

Conclusion

The job of a newly qualified staff nurse is challenging and different from that of a senior student. Whilst the roles of individuals vary, as do their needs, commonly the traditional initial training does not prepare the student adequately for her first staff nurse post. Therefore, most newly qualified nurses require further knowledge and development of skills, particularly in management and certain aspects of communication and interpersonal relationships. This book explores the nature of the staff nurse's role, the necessary knowledge basis and ways of enhancing skills.

References

Benner, P. (1984) *From Novice to Expert*, California: Addison Wesley Publishing Company.

Buckenham, M. A. (1988) 'Student nurse perception of the staff nurse role', *Journal of Advanced Nursing*, Vol. 13, pp. 662–70.

Claus, K. and Bailey, J. (1977) *Power and Influence in Health Care*, St. Louis: C. V. Mosby.

Davis, B. (1983) 'Student nurses' perceptions of their significant others', in Davis, B. (ed.), *Research into Nurse Education*, Beckenham, Kent: Croom Helm.

Davis, F. (1975) 'Professional socialization as subjective experience: the process of doctrinal conversion among student nurses', in Cox, C. and Mead, A. (eds.) *A Sociology of Medical Practice*, London: Collier-MacMillan.

Henderson, V. (1966) *The Nature of Nursing*, London: Collier-Macmillan

Henderson, V. (1979) 'Preserving the essence of nursing in a technological age', *Nursing Times*, Vol. 75, No. 47, pp. 2012–13.

Humphries, A. (1987) 'The Transition from Student to Staff Nurse', Unpublished BSc Thesis, Leicester University.

Kershaw, B. and Salvage, J. (Eds.) (1986) *Models for Nursing*, Chichester: John Wiley.

Kramer, M. (1974) *Reality Shock – Why Nurses Leave Nursing*, St. Louis: C. V. Mosby.

Lathlean, J., Smith, G. and Bradley, S. (1986) *Post-Registration Development Schemes Evaluation*, Kings College, University of London.

Matthewson, C. (1985) 'Student nurse–staff nurse: what is the difference?' in Sykes, M., *Licensed to Practice: The Role of the Staff Nurse*, Eastbourne: Bailliere Tindall.

Menzies, I. E. P., (1960) 'A case study in the functioning of social systems as a defence against anxiety', *Human Relations*, Vol. 13, pp. 95–121.

Moores, B. and Moult, A. (1979) 'Patterns of nursing activity', *Journal of Advanced Nursing*, Vol. 4, No. 2, pp. 137–49.

Pearson, A. (1983) *The Clinical Nursing Unit*, London: Heinemann Medical Books.

Pearson, A. and Vaughan, B. (1986) *Nursing Models for Practice*, London: Heinemann.

Roy, C. (1970) Adaptation: a conceptual framework for nursing, *Nursing Outlook*, Vol. 18, No. 3

Simpson, I. H., Back, K. W., Ingles, T., Kerckhoff, A. C., McKinney, J. C. (1979) *From Student to Nurse: A Longitudinal Study of Socialization*, Cambridge University Press.

Singer, E. J. and MacDonald, I. D. (1970) *Is Apprenticeship Outdated?* London: Institute of Personnel Management.

United Kingdom Central Council for Nursing, Midwifery and Health Visiting (1986) *Project 2000. A New Preparation for Practice*, London: UKCC.

Vaughan, B. (1980) The Newly Qualified Staff Nurse – Factors Affecting Transition, Unpublished MSc Thesis, University of Manchester.

Appendix: Synopses of two unpublished research studies of newly registered nurses

1.1 The newly qualified staff nurse: factors affecting transition
Barbara Vaughan, 1980

This study investigated the areas of the role that newly qualified staff nurses found satisfying, worrying and difficult, and the areas of their work for which they felt ill-prepared. It also identified the areas of their work that they found most different from their experiences as students.

The sample was of forty-three nurses who had been registered for three months from five schools of nursing within two separate Regional Health Authorities, and the research method used was a personally delivered questionnaire which incorporated the critical incident technique. The question-naire was divided into two parts – Part I posed general questions about qualifications, experience, shifts worked and so on, whereas Part II asked in detail about satisfying and worrying incidents, aspects of the role that were different from being a student, adequacy of preparation, amounts of time spent on specified aspects of the role (such as administration, direct clinical care, teaching), expectations and experiences, helps and hindrances. Thirty-eight completed questionnaires (including six from the pilot study) were analysed.

The majority of the respondents were female and aged between twenty and twenty-four years. The open responses relating to satisfying incidents were categorised (each person was asked to identify two), and five main categories were identified. In order of times mentioned they were: clinical; relationship with patients; management of the ward; relationship with staff; and teaching junior nurses. The responses related to worrying incidents (also two per person), in order of number mentioned, were: management; relations with staff; clinical; and relationship with patients/relatives. Four types of response relating to aspects of the role that were most different from being a student were found – altered relationships (82 per cent); increased responsibility (73 per cent); increase in administration (50 per cent); and loss of patient contact (13 per cent). (Percentages in brackets indicate the proportion of respondents mentioning this aspect.)

Respondents were asked to identify subjects that should be included in their general training. The list included: principles of management (87 per cent); behavioural sciences (24 per cent); counselling (21 per cent); teaching skills (8 per cent); and the opportunity to practise running the ward (40 per cent). In terms of difficulties experienced with the role, four main aspects were cited: delegation and co-ordination of work (55 per cent); staff relations (32 per cent); talking to relatives (18 per cent); and the management system in the hospital (8 per cent). The reasons given for these difficulties were: staff attitudes (42 per cent); inadequate preparation (40 per cent); insecurity (21 per cent); and lack of time (16 per cent). (Percentages in brackets indicate the proportion of respondents mentioning this aspect.)

Vaughan specified five items which respondents were asked to 'rank' in order of the amount of time they spent on them. The items were ward administration, communication with professionals, direct clincal care, supervising clinical care and teaching. The ranking varied greatly, indicating the great variation in the jobs of individuals. However, the results suggested that 'significantly more people spend the greater proportion of their time in communicating with other professionals and the least amount of their time in teaching either students, patients or relatives'.

In discussing the findings, Vaughan acknowledges the small size of the sample, but argues that the purpose of the study was to find out whether problems existed in the transition from student to staff nurse, not to isolate solutions to problems. She concludes by saying,

> the overall impression gained from the study is that, although there are some aspects of her role for which the newly qualified staff nurse is well equipped, there are other areas in which she feels ill prepared and inadequate. Little difficulty was expressed in clinical responsibilities which were found to be the most rewarding part of the staff nurse's role. However, problems related to management skills and interpersonal relationships recurred throughout the findings.

As a result, Vaughan tentatively recommends more attention to be given to the teaching of these skills both in basic training and following qualification.

Reference

Vaughan, B. (1980) The Newly Qualified Staff Nurse – Factors Affecting Transition, Unpublished MSc Thesis, University of Manchester.

1.2 The transition from student to staff nurse: a study of factors affecting newly qualified nurses
Anne Humphries, 1987

This study was almost identical to that of Vaughan (1980) in that it had the same aims, that is: 'to identify in which ways the new staff nurses' role differed from that of student nurses, and which aspects they found satisfying, worrying or difficult to fulfil', and it used a very similar tool for data collection. However, unlike Vaughan it was concentrated on nurses within one school of nursing (Oxfordshire) only.

The sample was of 104 nurses who had qualified from one school, and who had taken up their first staff nurse post in the same health authority. Data were collected using a questionnaire which incorporated the critical incident technique. The second, and main, part of the questionnaire, was identical to that of Vaughan. The first part of the questionnaire covered biographical and other general questions, but was slightly shorter than Vaughan's. Sixty-two completed questionnaires were analysed (a 61 per cent response rate). Whilst the majority of respondents were aged between twenty and twenty-four years, the proportion was slightly lower than in Vaughan's study – 80 per cent compared with 90 per cent.

The satisfying incidents were categorised in the same way as in Vaughan's study, and a very similar pattern emerged, with clinical incidents topping the list. However, the proportion of satisfying incidents identified as 'clinical' was lower than in Vaughan's study – 37 per cent compared with 46 per cent of total incidents cited. The picture emerging for worrying incidents was different, however, with those described as 'relationships with staff' being most prevalent (31 per cent of all) compared with 'management' incidents (forming 41 per cent of total) in Vaughan's study.

In Humphries' study the proportion of worrying incidents labelled 'clinical' was greater than in Vaughan's study (29 per cent and 17 per cent of all incidents respectively). Some care does need to be taken in interpreting these results, though, since although four out of the five categories used to describe the responses to the question about worrying incidents were the same for both studies, a fifth category, that of the 'system', was given as a separate category in Humphries' study and was absorbed into other categories in the Vaughan study. Nevertheless, an overall different pattern between the studies seems to be apparent, with relationships with staff and clinical issues being of most and almost equal concern in Humphries' study, and management issues being the major concern in Vaughan's study. This seems to indicate a slight shift in emphasis regarding the concerns of newly registered nurses.

In terms of the perceived differences between the staff nurses' and student nurses' roles, from a totally open question a remarkably similar list emerged to that found in Vaughan's study, with a further one added on, that of greater autonomy. The percentages of respondents who cited the differences did vary, though, between the studies as follows: altered relationships (50 per cent); increased responsibility (84 per cent); increase in administration (18 per cent); loss of patient contact (5 per cent); and the extra category, greater autonomy (8 per cent). Thus a much lower proportion of respondents in the Humphries' study than in Vaughan's study saw 'altered relationships' and 'increase in administration' as differences (50 per cent compared with 82 per cent and 18 per cent compared with 50 per cent respectively). Although 'increased responsibility' was cited by almost three-quarters of respondents in Vaughan's study, it was even more noticeable to respondents in Humphries' study, with 84 per cent of them specifically commenting on it. When respondents were asked which subjects or aspects should be included in their general training they mentioned: management practice (42 per cent); interpersonal skills (25 per cent): deeper knowledge base (16 per cent); and personal supervision and support (16 per cent).

It is interesting to note that a much higher proportion in Vaughan's study than Humphries' study cited 'management' (87 per cent compared with 42 per cent of respondents), and that 'the opportunity to practise running the ward', a commonly mentioned aspect in Vaughan's study, did not feature at all as a category in the Humphries' study. This may well reflect the differences between the programmes of general training that the two groups of respondents encountered. Humphries, for example, describes a final 'Professional Development' module, lasting sixteen weeks, which spans the period immediately prior to and after the final examination, and during which the nurse prepares for her Ward Management Practical Assessment. Though the programmes are not specifically described in the Vaughan study, many training programmes changed a good deal during the 1980s, and it is possible that the emphasis on professional development and management was not as great in 1980 as it was in 1987, the respective years for the two studies.

In terms of difficulties experienced with the role, the following were mentioned: delegation (26 per cent); increased responsibility (23 per cent); staff relations (21 per cent); teaching (16 per cent); and relations with relatives (13 per cent). It is interesting to compare these reponses with those of Vaughan's study. Whilst some of the same concerns were shown in both studies, for example delegation and staff relations, the proportions of respondents in the Humphries' study experiencing such difficulties were lower than in the Vaughan study (26 per cent compared with 55 per cent and 21 per cent compared with 32 per cent respectively). Some new difficulties were mentioned in the Humphries' study, notably increased responsibility and teaching. It seems from this that nurses are becoming increasingly conscious of their enhanced responsibility as staff nurses, and their teaching roles. (Percentages in brackets indicate the proportion of respondents mentioning this aspect.)

The reasons given for these difficulties were: role conflict (31 per cent of all respondents); staff relationships (27 per cent); inadequate preparation (26 per cent); and nurses' insecurity (18 per cent). Interestingly, in the Vaughan study, role conflict, that is, the nurse feeling a 'jack of all trades' and experiencing conflict when coping with clinical and management responsibilities, was not included at all as a category, yet it was mentioned by more respondents than any other aspect. Conversely, lack of time, which was given as a reason for difficulties found by some in the Vaughan study, was not mentioned in the Humphries' study.

A similar picture emerged overall in both studies in relation to the question about the proportion of time spent in different activities, in that there was considerable variation between individuals. However, 'significantly more nurses spent the greatest proportion of their time communicating with other professionals and direct patient care and less on teaching and paperwork'. (Out of sixty-two respondents, forty-seven ranked communication as their first or second most time consuming activity, and thirty-seven ranked direct patient care likewise, whereas only seven ranked teaching as their first or second most time consuming activity, and fourteen, ward administration (paperwork).

This sample was also relatively small, and the author recognised its limitations, while suggesting that the study aims were sufficiently met. Humphries concludes that though most satisfaction was gained from direct patient care many of the nurses felt unprepared for the sudden increase in management responsibility, finding it difficult and stressful. As a result of the study, Humphries recommended that students be attached to staff nurse mentors during their final professional development module since it was experience and the opportunity to practise under supervision that had, or would have, helped them most to adjust to their new role. She also suggested that greater emphasis be given in the final stages of training to the acquisition of skills of communication, stress coping mechanisms, leadership and assertiveness.

Reference

Humphries, A. (1987) *The Transition from Student to Staff Nurse*, Unpublished BSc Thesis, Leicester University.

2 Providing Clinical Care

BARBARA VAUGHAN

Introduction

At a very early stage in their education student nurses become involved with the provision of nursing care for patients and, after three years of hard work, this appears to be the one aspect of their job about which they feel both competent and confident (Vaughan 1980, Lathlean 1986, and Humphries 1987). In many ways this is commendable, since the essence of nursing is concerned with working directly with patients and helping them to achieve their goals. Indeed, this is the reason that most people enter nursing in the first place, which is reinforced by the findings of both Humphries and Vaughan. They suggest that a high proportion of the incidents which newly registered nurses find satisfying in their work are related to clinical practice (Humphries 36.5 per cent [$N = 115$] and Vaughan 45.6 per cent [$N = 68$] of responses). Some of the instances they quote are ones which are familiar to many nurses:

> Seeing a little baby who had received major surgery and been ventilated from birth – now feeding on her mother's lap and wearing normal clothes.
> (Humphries 1987)

> To 'special' a dying patient in his last few hours and be with him when he died peacefully and comfortably. (Vaughan 1980)

Unfortunately the reality of the situation is not as simple as it may appear at first sight, and to some extent the joy of gaining registration can be marred by the frustrations which many nurses feel in the first few months after they qualify. Several factors can be identified which contribute to such a situation. For example, it is not uncommon for newly registered nurses to find that a significant proportion of their time is spent in carrying out work which is not directly concerned with clinical care. They may be overwhelmed with administrative and organisational tasks which can consume a disproportionate part of their working day. Indeed, in the mid-1970s Moores and Moult (1979) found that staff nurses spent on average nearly 60 per cent of their time undertaking non-clinical aspects of work, the majority of actual care being delivered by either student nurses or unqualified members of the team.

Priority setting, delegation of work, negotiation and organisation become the order of the day with little time or thought to pay much attention to the continuing development of practice, the one area in which they profess to feel confident. Furthermore, since these other tasks are often carried out by fairly senior people, they gather an ethos of being more important than the direct delivery of nursing. This may all add up to a state where the provision of clinical care takes on a routinised pattern, one of safety where old familiar or ritualised actions are perpetuated (Walsh and Ford 1989), through lack of time and energy to consider alternative ways of practising.

The transition stage

Moving from one role to another at any level is, in itself, stressful. Responsibilities are inevitably different as, by the very nature of the change, expectations alter. Never is this more conspicuous than the change from being a student to being a staff nurse. One day students are protected by the colour of their uniform, and despite the fact that difficult demands are made there are also allowances. Once they don the uniform of a registered practitioner the situation is quite different since there are overt signs which indicate to all that they are qualified nurses.

There are some positive factors in this change, such as more attention being paid to their opinion by patients, doctors and other nurses, though this says little for the way in which students are treated. However, it also brings extra strains. Students will come to the newly registered nurse requiring help with planning care; visitors to the ward will expect them to be familiar with what is happening; doctors will expect them to be able to make administrative decisions such as whether a new patient can be accepted; and the nurse will feel she should know all the answers. In reality this is never the case. Nevertheless, some newly registered nurses do find it very hard to admit to the fact that they are not suddenly 'all things to all men'. Such demands are often difficult to respond to and time consuming, especially in the early days after qualification. Frequently, they appear to take up a disproportionate amount of time leaving little space for working directly with patients.

There is no doubt that many nurses do feel a high degree of conflict in this sort of situation with a wide variation between what they would like to be able to do and what they can actually achieve. In the American college-based system this feeling has been called 'Reality Shock', caused by the variance between the real and the ideal world (Kramer 1974). Some have suggested that this syndrome is not apparent in the United Kingdom owing to our apprentice-type training. However, Kramer (1967) suggests that British nurses do in fact suffer from a similar syndrome which she terms 'Reality Stress' and which she suggests may be more dangerous because it is more insidious in nature. In order to cope with such a situation Kramer suggests that nurses follow one of four paths, all of which have descriptive and memorable names. The options include the following:

- *Lateral arabesque* – taking a sideways step from the real world and retreating back into education, where they can hang on to the way they think nursing should be, foregetting how life really is. It may be that they take up teaching posts or that they become perpetual students, unwilling to face the responsibility of a clinical role. It must be added that comments such as these do not detract from the importance of continuing education provided there are sound reasons, arising out of practice needs, for the routes which are followed. Indeed, this is one aspect which is essential to the ongoing development of nursing, but inappropriate if it is merely used as an escape route from reality.
- *Organisation woman* – in this instance what becomes most important is an adherence to the rules and regulations of the organisation. Professional ideals are rejected as being idealistic and unacceptable in a 'real world'. What matters most of all is that the organisation runs smoothly. They have been termed the 'clip board brigade', filling in forms, worrying about uniforms and enforcing the rules and regulations. In many ways this is just as much of an escape route as those who take a lateral arabesque, since so much time may be spent on administrative functions that there is no space left for facing the need for practice development. This description may be a little harsh as any organisation has to be well managed and live within its budget. But it becomes questionable when the rules become so inflexible that there is no room left for the professional discretion of individual practitioners to be exercised, and organisation women usually provide an efficient, routinised and unimaginative service.
- *Rutters* – these are the people who have said 'a plague on both your houses' and have given up. They cannot face the fact that priorities have to be set, that there is not a bottomless fund to provide help, that compromises have to be made. Some leave nursing and find other work. Others just come to work, do as they are told and go home again with their pay packets. They can find no compromise between the way they would like things to be and the way things really are, so they deny that there is a problem.
- *Bi-cultural trouble makers* – this is perhaps an unfortunate name but these are the people who recognise that the work culture does have constraints which inevitably put limits on practice. However, rather than denying the difficulties, escaping or giving up, they seek ways of hanging on to what they believe to be right, and slowly but surely finding ways of introducing the

professional culture which they value to the real world. The development of practice is central to their work and while they will acknowledge the need for compromise while still being able to live with their own consciences, they will strive for what they believe to be right. Bi-cultural trouble makers sometimes 'rock the boat' but hopefully through assertive rather than aggressive means. For example, while they may challenge certain aspects of practice they will also offer alternative solutions rather than just complain about the status quo. Thus they can make a discreet but positive contribution to clinical care.

It is easy to recognise colleagues and friends in these descriptions. The question which has to be raised is which path each newly registered nurse will choose to follow. Furthermore, the confidence about clinical practice which is felt by many nurses when they first qualify may, in reality, be a two edged sword, lulling people into a false sense of security. Thus while they may start in the belief that the bi-cultural trouble maker is the person they would like to be, they may not recognise the need for further development of their own practice. Yet there is some evidence to suggest that, on registration, nurses are only at the first stage of becoming clinically competent.

From novice to expert

Benner (1984) undertook a research study of beginning and expert nurses to determine differences in their clinical performance and how they appraised situations. In her findings, Benner describes the newly registered nurse as a novice, one who is only just beginning to develop the expertise needed to give clinical care. She suggests that the very nature of the way people are moved from setting to setting throughout their training never gives them time to become familiar enough with the patterns of progress to become proficient, and that it takes several years, and passage through a series of stages, to become an expert. Time is needed to extend both formal and informal learning in order to recognise the limits of current knowledge; to identify both desirable and acceptable standards; to develop methods of monitoring these standards; to make use of current research and identify areas for further work, all of which are fundamental to the development of a quality nursing service.

The stages which Benner describes fall into five broad categories. Recognition of these phases can, to some exent, overcome the feelings of inadequacy which are often experienced in the early days after qualifying, as it becomes apparent that it is unrealistic to think that expert practice can be achieved straight away. The five phases she describes are as follows:

1. *The novice* – one who is new to a situation and therefore unable to draw on past experience in order to make decisions. Hence the only guidance available is, in Benner's words, 'the context free rules' which have been

learned. It is a situation which many nurses will recognise, the feeling that they must respond to everything but cannot work out what needs doing first and what can safely be left until later. This, Benner suggests, is because while they have learned a set of principles they are unable to move away from these until they have learned to make judgements about their relative importance.

2. *The advanced beginner* – one who starts to recognise 'aspects' which may influence decision making in a particular situation and take a more global view of the world. However, lack of experience makes it difficult at this stage to recognise the multiplicity of alternatives which can occur. For example, two patients may both assure the nurse that now is the time to hear more information about their future. Their meaning may be quite different, one seeking reassurance and the other wanting more detail in order to plan his future.

3. *The competent practitioner* – this is a stage at which the nurse begins to see the part she has to play in the long term and how her actions can contribute to future situations. Thus her plans of today take into account situations which may arise later. She is able to plan her work effectively for a longer period of time. One of the most important characteristics of a competent practitioner is the *way* she plans her work, taking time at the beginning of the day to assess all those for whom she will be caring, attending to immediate needs and prioritising for less urgent but nevertheless important work. When a nurse reaches the point at which she can suddenly seem to make sense of the world in which she works, and has a degree of control over it, she can be described as a competent practitioner. As Benner says, then she has 'a feeling of mastery and the ability to cope with and manage the many contingencies of clinical nursing' (Benner 1984).

4. *The proficient practitioner* – it is at this stage that the nurse has attained a 'bank' of past experience in order to draw on a repertoire of situations which may help her in differentiating between what is relevant to the immediate circumstances. She is able to view the situation as a whole and will often appear to be unaware of certain 'aspects' since to her they are dismissed as not relevant in this particular situation. This is the sort of nurse who many may suggest acts intuitively, though in reality this may not be the case. It is that she has used her past experience in many ways to be able to short-circuit the steps which the newer nurse must pass through in order to be able to work effectively. She is speedy and efficient yet retains her humanity. Because of her skill in recognising such things as the importance of getting the timing of an intervention as well as the content right, there may be occasions when her decisions appear inexplicable to the less experienced. Yet much can be learned from such a practitioner. As Benner suggests it is the small 'nuances' which she is able to recognise which become so important.

5. *The expert practitioner* – in Benner's words 'the expert nurse, with an enormous background of experience, now has an intuitive grasp of each situation and zeros in on the accurate region of the problem without wasteful consideration of a large range of unfruitful, alternative diagnoses and solutions.' This is the nurse who can recognise that there is a problem brewing before it becomes apparent to others. She is the one who will tell you to 'keep a special eye on Mrs Smith' and is nearly always right. She may well have difficulty in saying how she knew or recognised that changes were occurring before they were recognised by others. She often puts it down to years of experience which, Benner suggests, is probably right, since she is quite clear that this stage cannot be reached without such a background.

Benner considers that it is impossible for anyone who is new to a clinical unit to be an expert straight away, including not only those who are newly qualified but also those who have not worked in a particular setting before. Indeed, she suggests that it can take two to three years to reach the stage of proficiency and more to advance to become an expert. Perhaps these timings appear to be rather long but in many ways it would be arrogant and would devalue practice to think that such skill can be gained without time and experience. Such an understanding can bring comfort not only to those who look with a degree of envy at their more experienced colleagues and wonder if they can ever achieve such efficiency, but also has implications for the habit which is so common in nursing of moving nurses from one environment to another. It provides an excellent rationale, when planning the future, for making such decisions as when to move to another area of work as well as helping to acknowledge and value what is still to be learned in a particular setting.

Factors influencing care giving

It is not difficult to fall into the trap of thinking that finding time to work directly with patients is sufficient to ensure that the quality of nursing his high. Unfortunately, this is far from true. The manner in which clinical care is delivered is dependent on many broader issues which cannot be ignored if the wish is to develop clinical practice. It is very often lack of consideration of these fundamental issues which can cause so much anguish for clinical nurses since if their importance is not fully recognised and acknowledged, then it is easy to find conflict in practice. For example, if no standards are set, nurses cannot know whether or not they are achieving desirable levels of practice. Similarly, if nurses are not aware of the research which is relative to their practice, then they cannot be sure of the accuracy of the knowledge on which they base their decisions. These things, and many others, are the foundations of good clinical care and if they are ignored by any qualified nurse, regardless of her level in the organisation, then practice itself will suffer. Thus if a quality service is to be developed it is essential that the importance of the underlying issues is acknowledged.

Organising work

One such issue is the way in which nursing work is organised. Much attention has been paid to this subject in recent years and there has been a move away from the traditional task allocation system towards patient allocation and primary nursing. While there were advantages to the old system of allocating tasks – everyone knew what was expected of them, it was easy to see who was responsible for given areas of work, junior staff could be expected to get on which unchallenging work safely, and so forth; there were also several disadvantages – patients had to relate to a great many different nurses, it was difficult to get the timing right, and there was often a queue of people waiting to attend to one person. Rest could not be planned and work which was not allocated was nobody's responsibility and so was often neglected.

Primary nursing can be seen as the other end of a continuum of ways of organising nursing work. It is a system where one qualified nurse is responsible, and hence accountable for all the nursing which a named group of patients receive while their need for nursing continues. This does not mean that this nurse has to actually give all the care personally, although it is expected that she will be involved in care giving as often as possible. It does mean that she is responsible for ensuring that the care is given according to the pre-planned programme even in her absence. In fact this system mirrors the way in which most professional practitioners organise their work.

Manthey (1980) offers a very clear guide to primary nursing. She suggests that the following four basic principles hold:

1. 'allocation and acceptance of individual responsibility for decision making to one individual'. Thus when a patient is admitted a named nurse is assigned to decide what nursing is needed and how that care will be given, and she retains that responsibility throughout the patient's stay.
2. 'assignment of care by case method'. Work is allocated to a named person, rather than by task, and that person will give all care within her competence, or ensure that it is completed.
3. 'direct person to person communication'. The pyramidal line of communication through the senior nurse is replaced by direct links between the person giving care and people involved.
4. 'one person operationally responsible for the quality of care administered to patients on a unit twenty four hours a day, seven days a week'. Because care is planned and given by the same person for the greater part of the time, that person can monitor the quality of the service more effectively.

The advantages to the patient of such a system are evident. Continuity of care can be achieved. Because there is a named nurse caring for a named patient it is clear who is responsible for all areas of care whether they were identified initially or at a later date. It is possible to see longer-term outcomes and the effectiveness of different methods of treatment. The relationship between the patient and the nurse can develop to a greater level of understanding and so more insight can be gained into individual needs.

There are several books about primary nursing written by British authors (e.g. Pearson 1987, Wright 1990 and Ersser and Tutton 1991). While this method of nursing is proving rewarding for both patients and nurses, the move from traditional practice is not easy. Many nurses have commented on the stress which they experience in the early stages, although in McMahon's (1989) opinion it is not primary nursing itself which is more stressful but the change from one system of organising work to another. This is borne out by the fact that once a team of nurses has become used to the responsibility, few would revert to old ways. However, the areas which they seem to find particularly difficult during the transition are practising autonomously, accepting responsibility for their own work, and the closeness of the relationship which can develop between patient and nurse. Once these have been overcome the effort does appear to be worthwhile. Anecdotal evidence suggests that there is a much higher degree of job satisfaction, that the nurses are more motivated and give more of themselves to their work. Perhaps one comment from a patient expresses the potential of this system from a different perspective. Following the change to primary nursing her view was: 'they used to put a body in its clothes – now they get me dressed'.

Undoubtedly there is much greater opportunity to really get to know the person for whom the nurse is caring and offer a more personalised service. This is demonstrated further by such things as an increase in 'follow up' telephone calls from patients once they leave the nurse's care, often just to let them know how things are going; or that letters are addressed to the patient's 'own' nurse rather than always to the sister of the ward. These examples may seem small and simplistic yet they all build up to a picture which suggests both happier patients and happier nurses.

There follow five basic principles which are worth considering before launching into such a challenging move:

1. Who should be a primary nurse? The responsibility within this role is great and, bearing in mind the comments of Benner (1984), most people would agree that there is a need for some experience following qualification before becoming a primary nurse. After all this is the key clinical role and asking someone who has just qualified to step straight into it would be the same as asking a newly qualified doctor to take full responsibility for the medical needs of a patient.

2. What preparation is available or can be planned for those who will accept the responsibility of being a primary nurse? If it is acknowledged that this is an advanced clinical role then some thought must be given to the help which can be offered, both in assisting people to gain the skills and in providing support for them once in the role. Burns (1988), in describing the role of the associate nurse, says that experience of this role is a prerequisite to becoming primary nurse.

3. How will the move affect other nursing roles within the unit? The most important one, according to Manthey (1980), is that of the ward sister since much of her traditional work will be delegated to the primary nurse. However, this certainly does not mean that her work is no longer needed. Indeed, the importance of good management and leadership with this system of organising nursing cannot be overstated. Having implemented primary nursing, Burns (1988) found that the role of sister became one of adviser on clinical issues rather than major decision maker.

   It is also very important to give consideration to those who will be acting as 'associate nurses', the ones who maintain the care prescribed by the primary nurse in her absence. One primary nurse may act as another's associate when she is not on duty. Alternatively this may be a very rewarding role for part-time staff, who do not work sufficient hours to be primary nurses, newly registered nurses, enrolled nurses or those who do not wish to be primary nurses. Very little research work has been undertaken in relation to the role of associate nurses to date, though there have been attempts to clarify the role, such as that by Wilson (1990). It must be recognised, however, that the system does not work without them and their role is of equal importance to any other in the unit.

4. How will the move affect other health care workers in the unit? It is much easier to gain support from other people in the unit if they are involved from a very early stage in the planning of a move of this kind. Consideration must be given to the responsibilities and constraints which are placed on all people working in an organisation, and there are times when compromises have to be made in order to accommodate their needs. Furthermore, others will sometimes have certain expectations because they are more familiar with a traditional way of working. For example, the consultant may expect the sister to accompany him and other medical staff on the doctors' rounds, whereas with primary nursing it is more usual for the nurse who is looking after a particular patient, or group of patients, to join the round at the appropriate point. After all, that nurse will be far more aware of the most recent developments and needs of the patient she has been caring for than the sister who will have more of an overview.

5. How will administrative responsibilities be managed? For example, it is important to look at such things as the way in which the duty rota will be

planned and to identify people who will accept responsibility for such things as safe custody of drugs or maintenance of equipment. It may be appropriate to organise such work on a 'task' basis, since although this may not be an ideal way of allocating responsibility for patient care it can be a very effective method of ensuring that other aspects of work are not neglected.

These are just some of the issues which need to be considered before making a move to primary nursing. However, it is worth adding that many of those who have made the effort and are now practising within a primary nursing system have found the change immensely satisfying.

Developing the quality of care in the ward environment

Frameworks for practice

Each nurse is – or should be – interested in providing a high-quality nursing service to patients, yet defining what is meant by such a statement is not easy. The problem is that there is no single dimension to quality and it will mean different things to different people according to what they value or deem to be important. The situation becomes even more complex when it is recognised that some of the people with whom an individual works may, in fact, have value systems different from their own and may thus view quality in a different way. This is one of the factors which can potentially cause so much conflict in practice. For example, a general manager, who is responsible for the provision of a cost-effective service, may equate quantity with quality, suggesting that the number of people who pass through the service is an appropriate measure. An alternative view, which some doctors hold, is that cure can be equated with quality, again something which is easily seen and measured.

So what about nursing? If the clinical contribution of nurses is to be valued equally alongside that of other health care workers then it is necessary to say what the purpose of the nursing service is and how this can be achieved. This is one of the reasons why it is so important for each clinical unit to have a clear framework or model for practice which states what is valued, what the purpose of the service is and how that purpose can be achieved. Indeed, this may be one of the most influential criteria which a newly registered nurse would look for when deciding where to work.

It is not sufficient to say that 'nursing is caring', a view which is commonly put forward. In reality such a statement says nothing of what the purpose of that care is, so how can one know if it has been achieved? Neither is it necessary in the initial phases to move to working with a highly developed model of practice, such as that described by Orem (1980), Roy (1976) or many others. What is essential is a statement of beliefs about the service which is offered, since without such a statement one cannot begin to say whether or not this is a quality service. Wright (1986) offers a description of how one unit's staff developed a model of their own which matched the personal beliefs of those who worked there. This may be a path which other nurses choose to follow since it offers both freedom for the nurses to express their own views and the opportunity for creativity in their practice. However, it does have to be borne in mind that this is a complex and difficult thing to do and it may be easier to adapt a model which has already been well described to meet local needs. (Fig. 2.1 gives an example of a ward philosophy and its effect on practice.)

Fig. 2.1 The influence of philosophy on practice (Source: Vaughan and Pillmoor 1989)

Statement	Effect on practice
People	
1. Are biological creatures subject to disease	Assessment will only be concerned with biological functions and disease
2. Are holistic beings who function as a whole	Assessment will include social and psychological aspects
3. Should take the advice of experts	Patients/clients should be told what is the right course of action
4. Have a right to choose	Patients/clients are given sufficient information to choose alternative approaches to treatment (if they wish)
Health	
1. Is the absence of disease	Cure at all costs
2. Is feeling well and able to achieve those things which are important to the individual	Establish individual's desired level of 'wellness' which may/may not conform to health workers' views of health
Nursing	
1. Is caring for people	Nurses will provide care (do *for*)
2. Is helping people to care for themselves	Nurses will help people (when they can or wish) to care for themselves (do *with*)
3. Is primarily concerned with the patient as an individual	Will view the patient's family as a secondary concern (who have temporarily handed over care to nurses)
4. Is concerned with the patient as an individual who is part of a family and society at large	Will be concerned about how the family is affected by the patient's hospitalisation and help them (if they wish) to contribute to care

A statement of beliefs or philosophy is not something which should live in a drawer in the office and only be brought out for visits from the tutorial staff or the National Board officers. It should be a live document, one which can help each nurse to set priorities and assess where she is in terms of the quality of the service. It provides a basis to identify areas which could be measured in order to begin to identify strengths or weaknesses in practice. For example, suppose one believes in self-care or independence as a goal of nursing. It is an interesting exercise to review the care plans and see how many of the activities which are recorded are actually related to helping people to regain independence and how many are concerned with 'doing things for people'.

Similarly, assessment data can be reviewed to see if they actually reflect the views of people. If the belief is in holistic care, is there a balance between physical, social and psychological information recorded, or is the emphasis on the disease process and physiological data? It may be that this is appropriate for some patients who were so sick on admission that their personal priorities were only concerned with their own physical well-being. But if this is the regular pattern then questions should perhaps be raised about whether practice actually reflects what has been stated.

Standard setting

Using a statement of beliefs in this way can be seen as the beginning of setting standards. A standard is a statement of the practice which is expected in relation to a particular criterion or aspect of work. It is a subject which has gained much interest in the past few years and a great deal has been done to try to help people to start on the path of identifying standards of practice at both local and national levels (Kitson 1988 and 1989). What has become apparent is that the most appropriate place for clinical standards to be identified and set is within a ward or unit, where the staff who are actually involved with giving care can take part (Kendall and Kitson 1986).

Rather than trying to set standards for every aspect of work initially, some people have used this method as a way of tackling a specific problem (Howell and Marr 1988). For example suppose there is concern about the way in which patients are given their drugs prior to discharge. In terms of the statement of beliefs, if part of the nursing function is to help people to be independent then it is important that patients are familiar with handling their own drugs prior to going home. Thus a standard which reflects this belief may be agreed upon such as the following:

- Patients will receive their own drugs at least 24 hours prior to discharge.
- Prior to discharge, patients will be able to identify each drug, say what it is for, and know when and for how long it should be taken.

Setting standards of this kind makes the expectations quite explicit to all members of the nursing team. Furthermore, it gives clear grounds for negotiation with other members of the multidisciplinary team, should there be a need to negotiate the date of discharge.

Standard setting can also act as a very useful guide in relation to the job description and what is expected to the individual. For example, there is often a key result area which reads something like: 'Will maintain personal and professional development.' This is a common requirement of any employee, but may be viewed in different ways by different people, and if no guidance is given as to exactly what is meant, then it is difficult to know whether or not it has been achieved. It is possible to set standards which are more precise such as:

- Will read at least one professional journal regularly (time – ongoing);
- Will develop knowledge in relationship to catheter care (or other subject which is relevant to the clinical unit) and prepare a resource file for the ward (time three months).

These statements make clear the expectations and allow the achievement of this key area of the job to be evaluated.

Ideally these are the sorts of things which should be shared within the clinical team and be part of the ward's normal practice. In reality, though, this is not always the case. Even so, there is no reason why one or more team members cannot set personal standards related to personal progress which can act as an incentive to development. In this way clear goals to strive for can be set, and areas in which more work or support are needed can be identified, thus giving something more tangible to judge progress against. Robinson and FitzGerald (1990) describe a standard setting exercise that improved staff nurses' practice and their professional development.

Two words of warning must be added in relation to setting standards. First, it is of no value to set standards which are totally unattainable. This can lead to frustration and despondency for all concerned. Nevertheless, standards should reflect the professional values of nursing. Second, it is always worth remembering that nurses do not work in isolation and it is important to remember the contribution which other members of the team have to make when considering standards of nursing care. For example, it is of no help to set a standard related to flexible meal times if the domestic staff cannot also adjust their work. Similarly, consideration has to be given to such things as the fixed times when doctors have to attend out-patients or theatres, when considering the best way of maintaining interdisciplinary communication.

Resolving conflicts

One of the most valuable outcomes of having a unit philosophy and identifying standards is that it gives firm grounds for priority setting and negotiation. In any nurse's day there never seems to be enough time to do everything and decisions have to be made about what can be achieved realistically in the time available. Indeed, this is one of the greatest causes of stress to many nurses since, understandably, all would like to be able to given an 'ideal service'. But life is just not like that. What is important is that each nurse can go home at the end of the day in the knowledge that, given the time and resources available, the right decisions were made about what was done.

In circumstances such as these it is very easy to fall into the trap of doing 'visible' familiar work, especially when there seems so much to do that there is an urgency to 'get on with things'. However, if time is not taken at the beginning of the day to review the work needed, it is quite possible that the less obvious, but often more important work, may be left uncompleted because there is not enough time to do everything. For example, suppose there is the choice of spending some time with a patient who is going to theatre for major surgery the following day or making the beds. Bed making is visible and an easy task to fulfil. What is more, the nurse may be concerned that people will think she is inefficient if this task is not done. Spending time talking with a patient prior to surgery is invisible and much more difficult to do if it is to be of any value; other people may not be able to see easily that the work is done. Yet consider the outcome of having to leave either of these areas of work undone. The consequences of not giving pre-operative information are far-reaching since there is ample evidence to relate post-operative recovery to the giving of pre-operative information (see for example Hayward 1975; Boore 1978). The consequence of leaving beds unmade until later in the day may be seen at a nuisance level but does not have such severe outcomes.

This example may be a bit extreme since at the end of the day it is unlikely that the beds will be left unmade. However, it serves to show that it is much easier to do what can be seen, sometimes at the cost of less obvious but more important work. The 'action phase' of work takes priority over the 'thinking stage' and, just as with patient care, unplanned work can be unproductive. Thus in organising work and setting priorities there is an urgent need to plan. Furthermore, by relating the planning phase to the philosophy and standards which have been agreed to, it is easier to decide which work is most urgent. In this way, while it may still be frustrating not to be able to do everything, at least it will be possible to judge whether the decisions made were reasonable in the light of the circumstances.

A further value of being clear about the purpose of nursing work is that it helps to formulate ideas when contributing to multidisciplinary team work. One of the things which some nurses find difficult to cope with is the perceived power of doctors in decision making, without consideration being given to the things which they, as nurses, feel to be important. For example, Vaughan (1980) quotes an experience of one newly registered nurse who was very concerned by the decision of the medical team to withhold information from a patient about his diagnosis of carcinoma with a very poor prognosis. Yet the man concerned was a devout Catholic with a young family and she felt that he had a right to the chance of being told the truth, if that is what he wished. Other examples of this nature include such things as whether or not medical treatment should be continued, whether relatives' or patients' wishes should be followed (particularly in relationship to divulging difficult information) or indeed whether offers of help should be withdrawn if patients do not 'comply' in behaviour which is acceptable to those who are offering the service.

Such dilemmas are commonplace but are not easy to handle. If nurses are sure of their attitudes towards such things as human rights and truth telling, it is much easier to negotiate a unit policy involving the total team than if only emotive arguments are put forward. Furthermore, exploring the way in which moral views influence practice can help to show why it is that agreement cannot always be reached and that people do in fact hold differing views about such basic things as human rights. There is little doubt that the importance of the whole area of moral philosophy is one which has gained recognition in recent years and there are now several texts which deal with this subject (for example, Campbell 1984; Downie and Calman 1987).

Research

Recognition of the importance of research to nursing is relatively new and there is still a long way to go, not only in developing the knowledge base for practice, but also in making use of the available information. Essentially, at a clinical level what is needed is 'research mindedness' – a willingness to challenge current ideas and give careful thought to the rationale on which actions are based. It is unreasonable to expect every nurse to undertake research personally. What *is* reasonable is that every nurse should be aware of current information about her field of practice.

There are many ways of increasing research awareness at a clinical level such as starting a journal club, collating files of current articles about relevant areas of practice, challenging traditional practice through care conferences or reviewing care plans. However, not all research which has been undertaken is applicable generally; neither is all research well done. It is therefore very important for all nurses to have a fundamental understanding of the research process in order to be able to make a judgement about whether work is both acceptable and relevant to their area of practice. Unfortunately, this is not a skill which is always incorporated into initial nurse education. There are opportunities for nurses to increase their understanding of the research process through formal courses, such as the Diploma of Nursing or others approved by the National Boards, through attending locally organised study days. workshops and seminars, or through the use of distance learning materials (see, for example, the *Distance Learning Centre Research Series*).

While the importance of research cannot be overestimated, acceptance of experience, personal growth and intuitive practice should not be forgotten either. Nursing has been described as both a science and an art, and if emphasis is given purely to the scientific perspective there is a risk that the artistry of practice may suffer. Carper (1978) suggests that the knowledge on which practice is based is derived from four basic sources, namely empirical evidence (the science), aesthetics (the art), personal knowledge of self and moral knowledge or awareness of how our moral judgements may influence the way of working. It is the *manner* in which all these things are put together which is so important. Fig. 2.2 shows just one example of the differing sources of knowledge which may be drawn on in a relatively common clinical situation – administration of a prescribed drug.

Fig. 2.2   Sources of knowledge

Situation – administration of a prescribed drug
- Empirical knowledge – related to such things as the dosage, factors which may influence the absorption, and side-effects.
- Aesthetic knowledge – which may be concerned with helping someone to swallow a large pill, disguising unpleasant tastes and the manner in which the patient is approached.
- Personal knowledge – may be related to one's own like/dislike of taking medicine or the way the nurse feels about giving drugs which are known to have unpleasant side-effects such as can be the case with cytotoxic therapy.
- Moral knowledge – may raise issues about how the nurse should respond if someone does not wish to take his medication or indeed if it is felt that the drug which has been prescribed is inappropriate in this particular situation.

Recognition of all these aspects can broaden the perspective of the way of working on a day-to-day basis, as well as giving some insight into how practice is developed. It is of little value to gain a deeper understanding of pharmacology if in the end it is not possible to help someone to swallow pills. Furthermore, the way in which the nurse reacts, especially if she is unhappy about some aspects of administering a particular drug, will inevitably have an effect on the patient.

There are times in practice when all nurses act 'intuitively' because they feel that something is right. With the advent of science in nursing it has been suggested that intuition is neither acceptable nor safe. Yet it can be argued that intuition arises from an accumulation of all that is known or learnt over a long period of time, even if it is difficult to bring that 'knowing' to the surface. Schön (1983) argues that this so-called intuitive practice of experts is a skill to be valued and suggests that through reflecting on practice itself and what he calls the 'used rather than the espoused (taught or recommended) knowledge', much insight and understanding can be gained (this is discussed further in Chapter 5). One way of doing this at a personal level may be through keeping a journal or diary and recording both satisfying and worrying incidences and 'reflecting' on why they happened and the knowledge used when decisions were made. At times this may demonstrate the deficits which everyone has in some areas of knowledge and give direction to enquiry. It may also help to bring to the surface that intuitive knowledge which can then be shared with others. Furthermore, this may be the beginning of taking research in practice the next stage on from awareness to small-scale enquiry at a clinical level since the most pertinent questions so often arise out of practice itself.

Broadening clinical skills

Developing new clinical skills and incorporating them into practice can be one of the most rewarding experiences for any nurse. While there are many specialist skills related to the technical aspects of health care which it may be appropriate for nurses to learn, this is not the only direction in which they may choose to develop. The introduction of primary nursing may lead to a need to understand more about autonomous practice and the therapeutic relationship which can develop between patient and nurse. The need to manage a clinical case load may demand a greater understanding of priority setting and time management. The choice of directions is endless but since no one can be an expert in all fields it is important to find the type of learning which would be of greatest benefit in the particular field in which the nurse works.

   One interesting path which some nurses have chosen to follow is in learning to practise a so-called 'complementary therapy'. As the importance of holistic care is becoming more widely recognised a wealth of opportunities is opening for nurses to extend their skills in less traditional, but often much older, forms of therapy. There are many examples of these sorts of skills which some patients also find much more acceptable than the use of drugs or other more invasive treatments. For example, many nurses are now learning the basic skills of massage which they find invaluable in helping patients with symptoms which do not always respond well to more conventional treatments, such as pain, sleeplessness, constipation or anxiety. Foot massage has been found to be particularly beneficial with elderly patients (Thomas 1989). Acquiring a sufficient understanding of massage to help patients is not difficult and opportunities to learn are becoming more available in many areas (see Trevelyan 1989).

Therapeutic touch is another technique which has recently attracted interest (Smith 1990). The importance of touch in non-verbal communication has long been recognised and the use of touch by nurses has been encouraged and investigated widely (LeMay and Redfern 1987). Many nurses see it as a logical step to use touch as an intervention to help relieve tenseness and a variety of other symptoms in patients. Again this is a non-invasive therapy which can being relief to some patients and the closeness of nurses with patients offers an ideal entry to this form of help (Wyatt and Dimmer 1988).

Herbal remedies and dietary changes are other areas which have been explored and found to be helpful by both patients and nurses (Passant 1990). Aromatherapy has been used on many different types of ward to relieve anxiety, encourage sleep and to aid analgesia (Tisserand 1988; Wise 1989). Aromatherapy is the use of 'essential' oils concentrated from plants to promote well-being. The oils can be added to bath-water, evaporated using a fragrancer or used in a variety of other ways. One of the most common ways of using the essence is to add a few drops to oil being used for massage. Relaxation, shiatsu (acupressure), yoga, tai chi and reflex zone therapy (Evans 1990) are other examples of skills which some nurses have incorporated into their practice, in many cases taking advantage of their new found knowledge for both themselves and the patients with whom they work.

Conclusion

Providing good clinical care for patients is both the most rewarding and the most demanding part of any nurse's role. However, the provision of such care is dependent on a myriad of different factors and goes beyond just 'doing'. Careful thought has to be given to all the underlying factors which help ensure that the quality of the service offered meets the demands of both the patients and the practitioners. If there is no framework there will be no clearly defined direction. If standards are not set there can be no way of knowing if they have been achieved. If knowledge is not expanded then practice can become routinised and complacent.

As with any other occupational group the point at which a professional nursing qualification is gained can only be the beginning of the path towards becoming an expert practitioner. Recognition of learning needs and a commitment to continue developing throughout the rest of the nurse's career are hallmarks of professional practice and ones which, it is hoped, all nurses will demonstrate. This is not an easy challenge to take up. There are times when the energy required to learn new methods and incorporate new skills into practice is difficult to find. The provision of clinical care for patients is the central focus of all nursing work and, at the end of the day, the satisfaction which can be felt in knowing that a job has been well done is well worth all the effort.

References

Benner, P. (1984) *From Novice to Expert*, California: Addison Wesley Publishing Company.

Boore, J. R. P. (1978) *Prescription for Recovery*, London: Royal College of Nursing.

Burns, S. (1988) 'The role of the associate nurse', *The Professional Nurse,* Vol. 4, No. 1, pp. 18–20.

Campbell, A. (1984) *Moral Dilemmas in Medicine*, 3rd. ed., London: Churchill Livingstone.

Distance Learning Centre (1988 onwards) *Research Series*, Polytechnic of the South Bank.

Carper, B. (1978) 'Fundamental patterns of knowing in nursing', *Advances in Nursing Sciences*, October Vol. 1(1), pp. 13–23.

Downie, R. S. and Calman, K. C. (1987) *Healthy Respect*, London: Faber and Faber.

Ersser, S. and Tutton, E. (eds.) (1991) *Primary Nursing in Perspective*, London: Scutari Press.

Evans, M. (1990) 'Reflex zone therapy for mothers', *Nursing Times*, Vol. 86, No. 4, pp. 29–31.

Hayward, J. (1975) *Information: a Prescription Against Pain*, London: Royal College of Nursing.

Howell, J. and Marr, H. (1988) 'Raising the standards: visible improvement,' *Nursing Times*, Vol. 84, No. 25, pp. 33–4.

Humphries, A. (1987) *The Transition from Student to Staff Nurse*, Unpublished BSc Thesis, Leicester University.

Kendall, H. and Kitson, A. (1986) 'Rest assured', *Nursing Times*, Vol. 82, No. 35, pp. 29–31.

Kitson, A. (1988) 'Raising the standards,' *Nursing Times*, Vol. 84, No. 25, pp. 28–32.

Kitson, A. (1989) *A Framework for Quality: A Patient-centred Approach to Quality Assurance in Health Care*, London: Royal College of Nursing.

Kramer, M. (1967) 'Comparative study of characteristics, attitudes and opinions of neophyte British and American nurses'. *International Journal of Nursing Studies*, Vol. 4, pp. 281–94.

Kramer, M. (1974) *Reality Shock – Why Nurses Leave Nursing*, St Louis: C. V. Mosby.

Lathlean, J., Smith, G. and Bradley, S. (1986) *Post-Registration Development Schemes Evaluation*, Kings College, University of London.

LeMay, A. C. and Redfern, S. J. (1987) 'A study of the non-verbal communication between nurses and elderly patients', in Fielding, P. (ed.) *Research in the Nursing Care of Elderly People*, Chichester: John Wiley.

McMahon, R. (1989) 'Partners in care', *Nursing Times*, Vol. 85, No. 8, pp. 34–5.

Moores, B. and Moult, A. (1979) 'Patterns of nurse activities', *Journal of Advanced Nursing*, Vol. 4, No. 2, pp. 137–49.

Orem, D. (1980) *Nursing – Concepts of Practice*, 2nd edn, New York: McGraw Hill.

Pasant, H. (1990) 'A holistic approach in the ward', *Nursing Times*, Vol. 86, No. 4, pp. 26–8.

Pearson, A. (ed.) (1987) *Quality Assurance*, London: Croom Helm.

Robinson, K. and FitzGerald, M. (1990) 'Setting standards: a staff-centred approach'. *Nursing Times*, Vol. 86, No. 14, pp. 42–3.

Roy, C. (1976) *Introduction to Nursing – An Adaptation Model*, Old Tappan, New Jersey: Prentice Hall.

Schön, D. A. (1983) *The Reflective Practitioner – How Professionals Think in Action*, London: Temple Smith.

Smith, M. (1990) 'Healing through touch', *Nursing Times*, Vol. 86, No. 4, pp. 31–2.

Thomas, M. (1989) 'Fancy footwork', *Nursing Times*, Vol. 85, No. 41, pp. 42–4.

Tisserand, R. (1988) 'Aromatherapy on the wards', *International Journal of Aromatherapy*, Vol. 1, No. 2, p.8

Trevelyan, J. (1989) 'Relaxing with massage', *Nursing Times*, Vol. 85, No. 39, pp. 52–3.

Vaughan, B. (1980) The Newly Qualified Staff Nurse – Factors Affecting Transition. Unpublished MSc Thesis, University of Manchester.

Vaughan, B. and Pillmoor, M. (1989) *Managing Nursing Work*, Chichester: John Wiley.

Walsh, M. and Ford, P. (1989) *Nursing Rituals, Research and Actions*, Oxford: Heinemann Nursing.

Wilson, K. (1990) 'An associate in care', *Nursing Times*, Vol. 86, No. 42, pp. 63–4.

Wise, R. (1989) 'Flower power', *Nursing Times*, Vol. 85, No. 22, pp. 45–7.

Wright, S. G. (1990) *Building and Using a Model of Nursing*, London: Arnold.

Wright, S. G. (1990) *My Patient – My Nurse; the Practice of Primary Nursing*, London: Scutari Press.

Wyatt, G. and Dimmer, S. (1988) 'The balancing touch', *Nursing Times*, Vol. 82, No. 21, pp. 40–3.

3   Managing the Ward and Nursing Work

ANGELA HESLOP AND JUDITH LATHLEAN

Introduction

Being in charge of a ward is a common experience for many new staff nurses. In their research on newly registered nurses, Lathlean *et al.* (1986) found that half of the newly registered nurses they studied had taken total charge of their wards within the first month following registration, and the majority were regularly in charge during the first six to nine months. Humphries (1987) found that 98 per cent of her sample had taken charge of the ward on occasions, with almost a quarter reporting that 'they were frequently left in charge despite the acute nature of the wards and [their own] inexperience'. A rather higher proportion of the nurses in Vaughan's (1980) research – nearly 60 per cent – were often in charge.

What are the feelings of new staff nurses about being left in charge of the ward and making decisions in relation to ward management? Both Vaughan's (1980) and Humphries' (1987) studies asked newly registered nurses to describe the two most satisfying and worrying incidents that had occurred to them, in the first study, during the previous six months, and in the second, since completing their training. Vaughan found the highest number of worrying incidents were about being in charge and ward management (almost a quarter of all worrying incidents mentioned); Humphries found less (almost 17 per cent). Typical problems cited were:

> The day after I received my certificate for SRN I was left in charge. One minute I was a student, the next a staff nurse. That day we had two ward rounds, four admissions, three discharges and a death. I was extremely worried . . . as I wondered if I would cope. Thankfully I did because I knew the routine as a student in that ward. If it had been a new ward I wouldn't have been able to.
>
> (Vaughan 1980, p. 121)

> Being the only trained member on duty. It was my first day as a staff nurse.
>
> (Humphries 1987, p. 104)

Conversely, being in charge and managing was found by some nurses to be satisfying:

> [I found it satisfying] the first shift when I was in charge and coped well with several dramas. I knew what to do and people appeared to have confidence in me.
> (Humphries 1987, p. 102).

> Being left in charge for the first time and actually being able to cope with the situation [was satisfying].   (Vaughan 1980, p. 119)

It seems that the factors influencing whether the experience of managing was good or bad – satisfying or worrying – include having the knowledge of what to do, having confidence and a belief that others, too, are confident in oneself, and actually getting through the experience without anything going disastrously wrong. Knowledge and confidence come in large part from education and practice, aspects which are often noticeably lacking in the three years' training where 'little time is devoted to the acquisition of skills related to management or teaching' (Vaughan 1980). The need for development of knowledge and skills in ward management was identified in Lathlean *et al.*'s (1986) study where it was concluded that 'for most newly registered nurses this appears to be the major issue concerning them in their first few months as a qualified nurse'.

This chapter looks at management – the skills and activities involved, and the practical issues that nurses need to tackle. It is difficult and perhaps artificial to separate out the role of the nurse as manager and that of provider of clinical care, communicator and teacher. Therefore, some of the important aspects of managing are also discussed elsewhere, particularly in Chapters 2, 4 and 5.

The newly registered nurse as manager

The newly registered nurse may not feel that she is a manager, nor that she wants to be involved with management or administrative activities at the expense of caring for patients. Some would identify the sister/charge nurse as the first level of manager, not seeing that they too have to 'manage' in order to be effective carers.

Managing the ward cannot and should not be separated from managing nursing work on an individual or team basis. In fact, the activities of nursing management and providing clinical care for patients should be thought of as part of a continuum, as shown in Fig. 3.1. The activities on the far left (A) describe the usual role of student or, with primary nursing (see Chaper 2), the associate nurse. Most newly registered nurses are likely to move between B and C, whereas the sister/charge nurse operates mainly in mode D. Ideally, the new nurse should be allowed to move gradually from the left-hand side of the continuum to the right, with a gradual increase of responsibility. The reality of many wards is that the newly registered nurse is often the most senior nurse on duty and has to take charge. Both Lathlean *et al.*'s (1986) study and Humphries' (1987) study included some nurses who, by the end of their first six months in post, were the most experienced RGNs on their ward.

Fig. 3.1   The management of nursing: a continuum

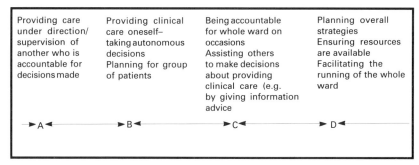

The newly registered nurse's role in 'managing' includes management of the whole ward, managing a team, managing a group of individual patients and managing themselves. Table 3.1 illustrates some of the most important aspects of each.

Table 3.1   The newly qualified nurse's role as manager

Managing the ward	Managing the team and individual patients	Managing oneself

The structure:
  unit profile
  organisation of patients' day
  organisation of nurses' day
Organising the nursing team
Skill mix and off-duty
Budgeting and resource control
Control of the physical
  environment
Health and safety at work
Management of standards
	Sharing administrative jobs
	
	Managing patient care:
	  individual patient need
	    assessment
	  clinical management
	
	Discharging a patient home
	
	Patients' rights
	
	Ethical considerations
		Managing the transition
		
		Time management
		
		Managing stress

The principles of management and the question of what is effective management have been studied extensively. A consideration of some of the ideas about management in general is a useful starting point for an understanding of the managerial aspect of the nurse's role.

What is management?

Managing the ward is a process whereby the skilled nursing of patients is facilitated, with attention to effectiveness and efficiency. Good management should help nurses to care for their patients. So whether the nurse is involved in management of the whole ward or is trying to manage her own workload, certain principles and activities are important.

Approaches to management

There is no one theory of management as such. Rather, there are a number of views about management and the way that organisations, and the people within them, work. At the beginning of the century a common view was that money was the main determinant of how hard and how well people worked. People were considered to be inherently lazy and motivated either by the desire for money or the fear that it would be withdrawn. The 'carrot and stick' approach to management was prevalent – that people can be encouraged by financial rewards and punished by them being withheld. This view was strongly challenged by the social scientists who conducted research into what motivates people at work, particularly as a result of the 'Hawthorne Experiment', conducted in the 1920s (summarised by Schein 1965). In this study, the physical conditions of women working in a company assembling telephone equipment were varied, but, whatever changes were made, output increased. The conclusion was reached that the women were responding to the greater attention that they were receiving.

Subsequently, Maslow (1954) defined a hierarchy of people's needs – physiological, safety, social, self-esteem and self-realisation – showing the value and importance of satisfying 'higher' needs, such as social and self-esteem, in work settings. Around the same time, another researcher, Herzberg (1966), studied those factors that affect levels of satisfaction and dissatisfaction at work and decided that they were not simple opposites, but were to be found in different aspects of the work. Dealing with the dissatisfying factors does not turn them into satisfying or motivating factors. In general, the dissatisfying factors – which he labelled *hygiene* or *maintenance* factors – were to do with conditions of work: company policy and administration; supervision; salary; interpersonal relations; and physical working conditions. He argued that these were the necessary conditions of successful motivation. The satisfiers – referred to as *motivators* – were identified as achievement; recognition; work itself; responsibilty; and advancement. Good hygiene is concerned with the question 'Why work here?' and the motivators with 'Why work harder?' This has obvious implications for nursing and management – it is insufficient to attend solely to working conditions; attention must also be paid to the motivators in achieving good work. So, for example, the dissatisfaction expressed by many nurses about clinical grading was not necessarily to do with the desire for more money. It was also related to their feelings that their worth was not sufficiently recognised by managers and that the actual work they were doing was being devalued by the managers.

McGregor (1960), convinced that management practices were more complex than had been described, took a different starting point by concentrating on the *nature* of people. He put forward two sets of propositions about human nature known as Theory X and Theory Y.

Theory X assumes that the average person:

- is by nature lazy;
- lacks ambition, dislikes responsibility and prefers to be led;
- is self-centred and indifferent to needs beyond him/herself;
- is resistant to change;
- is gullible and not very bright.

This is very much in line with the previously mentioned 'carrot and stick' approach and means that the main task of managers is to motivate and control people; people must be persuaded, rewarded, punished and controlled and their activities directed.

On the other hand Theory Y assumes that:

- people are not by nature passive or resistant; if they are it is because of experiences they have had in the organisation;
- control and punishment are not the only way to make people perform well; a person is capable of self-direction if he/she is committed to the goals of the organisation;
- the motivation and potential for development are present in all; it is the responsibility of management to release this potential by arranging conditions so that people can best achieve their own goals by directing their own efforts towards the objectives of the organisation;
- with the right environment most people can learn to accept and also to seek personal responsibility.

McGregor did not see these two theories as different ends of a continuum but, rather, as two approaches to management. It is possible in nursing today to see evidence of both these approaches, but do they both work? Certainly the changes desired in nursing – for example, the development of nursing as a profession and the move toward greater autonomy and accountability for the nurse – can only really flourish if Theory Y approach is pursued.

Much research has also been undertaken on the nature of leadership; for example what are the characteristics of a good leader and what are the different styles of leadership?

By 1950 there had been over 100 studies of what makes a good leader, but the results lacked consistency, with only 5 per cent of the traits identified being common throughout. However, Handy (1985) suggests that, overall, most studies single out the following four characteristics:

1. *Intelligence*: above average though not of genius level. Particularly good at solving complex and abstract problems.
2. *Initiative*: independence and inventiveness, the capacity to perceive the need for action and the urge to do it. (Appears to correlate quite well with age, i.e. drops off after 40.)
3. *Self-assurance*: implies self-confidence, reasonably high self-ratings on confidence and aspiration levels, and on perceived ultimate occupational level in society.
4. *The helicopter factor*: the ability to rise above the particulars of a situation and perceive it in its relation to the overall environment.

Attention has been paid to different styles of leadership. The styles usually compared are the authoritarian and the democratic; the former normally entails leader control and decision making and the latter group control, participation and delegation. A third type is sometimes added – that of *laissez-faire* leadership, though some would argue that this is not a style of leadership but, rather, a lack of leadership (Lippitt and White 1958).

If a nurse in charge of the ward takes an authoritarian approach, she would decide herself what each member of the team should do, tell them and then monitor whether or not they did it properly. The directions would come from her as manager of the ward. If, however, a democratic style were operating, she would probably call a meeting of the team together, listen to all the views and then base her decision about who does what on the majority view. The action chosen is much more likely to be the result of a consensus. A nurse operating n a *laissez-faire* way would tend not to lead but, rather, to expect all the team members to get on with the work as best they could with little or no guidance from herself.

One might be tempted to conclude that democratic leadership is always preferable, but it has been shown that some people prefer to be led or directed, and in repetitive or routine work an autocratic or structured style of leadership can lead to higher productivity in the short term, though sometimes at the expense of staff morale. Also, there are times when a more directive type of leadership is needed, for example in a crisis or high stress situation such as a major accident or a cardiac arrest. Thus different styles of leadership can be appropriate in different circumstances. In conclusion, it is now considered that style alone is not the answer to effective leadership. Also important are the preferences of individuals working under the leader, the job in hand and the environment or setting.

While most of the research on management and leadership has been in industrial settings, there has been some interesting work which has highlighted the ward sister's leadership or management style. Fretwell (1982) found that a good learning environment was fostered by a democratic style of leadership, and Smith and Redfern (1989) similarly concluded that students judged as favourable sisters (and trained staff) who allowed students to be involved in decision making. On the other hand, Ogier (1982) found that change and innovation was more likely to occur if the sister was directive. This seems to confirm that different situations require different approaches.

Management is about making the best use of the resources available to meet certain ends or objectives. And, as described earlier, it can refer to the whole ward, to a patient group managed by a team leader or a named nurse or to the nurse alone. Each of these areas is now considered.

Managing the ward

Although the newly registered nurse may only take charge of the ward occasionally and may feel that ward management is more the province of the sister or senior staff nurse, she too has an important part to play. There are many considerations and aspects involved; this chapter will only touch on a few of the most relevant ones and the reader is strongly advised to look to the references and the section on further reading for additional guidance.

The ward manager, whether this be the sister/charge nurse or the nurse who has the responsibility for co-ordinating the ward for a particular shift, needs to make the best use of the resources that are available. The main resources are time, nursing staff, equipment and the ward itself. This is illustrated in Fig. 3.2. A unit (or ward) profile and a statement of the philosophy can provide a useful framework for the management of the ward and the nursing work.

A unit profile and ward philosophy

A unit profile is 'a description of the various aspects of the work of a ward which can be used to inform nurses, other members of the health care team, patients and their relatives; it may contain anything that can be justified as being informative and useful' (FitzGerald 1989). Most wards do not have a comprehensive profile but some are beginning to develop a collection of essential components, such as the staffing, the unit/ward's philosophy of care (including reference to a model of nursing used on the unit/ward) and opportunities for staff development. A unit profile can be a source of support to the relatively inexperienced nurse faced with the daunting task of being in charge of the ward, because it gives guidance on the direction in which the ward should be going as well as the commonly held beliefs and information about resources.

Fig. 3.2   Making effective use of resources in the ward (Adapted from Matthews 1987)

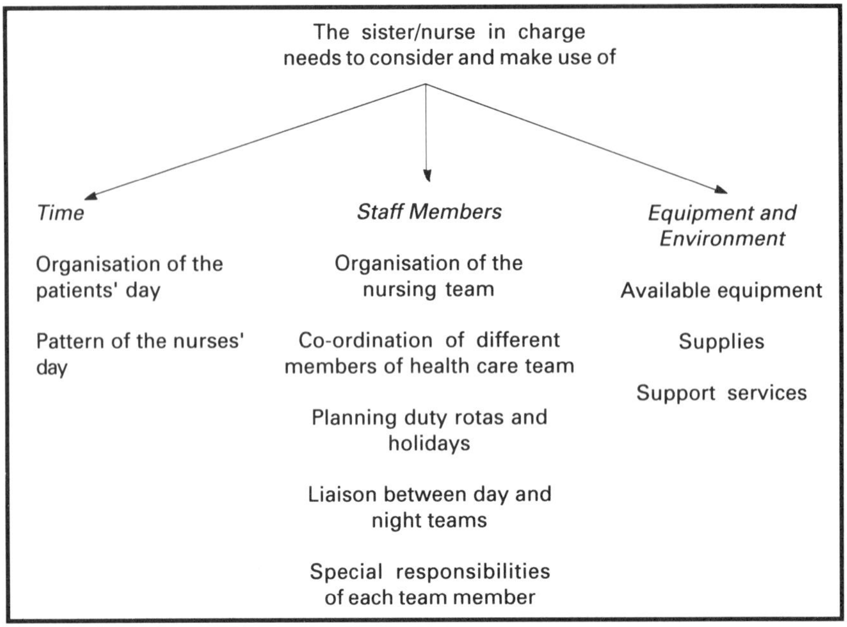

The sister/nurse in charge
needs to consider and make use of

Time	*Staff Members*	*Equipment and Environment*
Organisation of the patients' day	Organisation of the nursing team	Available equipment
Pattern of the nurses' day	Co-ordination of different members of health care team	Supplies
		Support services
	Planning duty rotas and holidays	
	Liaison between day and night teams	
	Special responsibilities of each team member	

How the ward sets out to achieve day-to-day working targets is influenced by its philosophy of care (a vital part of any unit profile), and this is reflected in the way nursing is organised. While nursing is unlikely ever to be totally independent of medical diagnosis and prescription, nurses have become increasingly interested in a professional model of practice. This is explicit or implicit in many ward philosophies. If the ward or unit does not have a written philosophy, that is, 'a concise statement of the nurses' attitudes, values and beliefs about issues which they consider important' (FitzGerald 1989), then steps can be taken to generate one. Fig. 3.3 gives one possible approach.

An example of a ward philosophy – and its potential effect on practice – is given in Chapter 2. The philosophy can be an important determinant of, or at least an influence on, many aspects of the ward's nursing work – the pattern of the patients' and nurses' day; the organisation of nursing work and nursing teams; the staff mix; the importance attached to and opportunities allowed for staff development and so on. (For further discussion of unit profiles and ward philosophies see FitzGerald 1989.)

The organisation of the patient's day

Much has been said and written about the pattern of the inpatient's day, but, with the increasing emphasis on planning individual patient care, attempts have

Fig. 3.3   Preparing a ward nursing philosophy of care

Finding out others' commitment:
- A ward philosophy should be the collective views of all members of the nursing team; therefore, the desire of all the nurses to be involved in its generation should be explored.

Gathering information:
- The presence of existing written philosophies in the hospital and health authority should be checked to avoid 'reinventing the wheel', to minimise potential conflict and to make use of other people's ideas.
- Reference should be made to documents expressing views about the role of the nurse or the standards of care that should be aimed for (e.g. UKCC Professional Code of Conduct; RCN's position statement on nursing).

Exploring different beliefs:
- The nursing team needs to decide which issues are to be included in the statement: 'Common choices are: the nature of people and human rights; methods of nursing; nursing goals; communication; the nature of health; education' (Fitzgerald 1989).
- Time should be set aside to discuss different views and reach an agreed consensus. Different methods can be used, e.g. by running a series of seminars; by choosing a sub-group to undertake preliminary work and report back to a meeting of all; by using a 'quality circle' (see p. 60); by individuals making written contributions which are collated by one or more persons.

Testing out the philosophy:
- Before using the philosophy as a basis for managing care on the ward, the document can be shared with other members of the multi-disciplinary team, to test that there are no potential conflicts or important aspects that have been overlooked. At the end of the day, however, the *nursing* philosophy adopted is the decision of the nurses.

---

been made to make the day more flexible and more related to individual needs and preferences. Nevertheless, in planning the patient's day many factors have to be considered such as any policies laid down by the hospital, services provided by other departments, and drug rounds. It may be impossible to alter the pattern of the day greatly because of the effect this has on others who are also contributing to the care of the patient, but sometimes factors which are thought to be sacrosanct, such as the time at which patients are expected to eat their meals, and even drug rounds, can be challenged and reviewed if it is in the best interest of the patient. For example, in the past, most patients have been habitually woken at 6.30 a.m. or even earlier, more for the convenience of the staff than that of the patients. Now, by careful discussion and negotiation between those involved, many wards do not wake patients until at least 7 a.m. or later.

Matthews (1987) gives an example of a patient's day which can be adapted to suit the requirements of individual wards. The newly qualified nurse will soon get to know the routine of her ward, but she is often in an ideal position to question the existing pattern if it seems not to be in the best interests of her patients. Of course there may be an unavoidable reason for it, but an open and flexible sister should welcome the fresh insights brought by the new nurse.

The organisation of the nurse's day

The pattern of the nurse's day is determined in part by the shift system of the hospital, but during the shift, it is greatly affected by the way that the nursing work is organised on the ward. Although there have been some challenges to the shift system, and there are exceptions to it, most wards find that adequate staff coverage and handover is best achieved by overlapping shifts of nurses. However, particularly in the light of the future shortage of nurses and the need to make it more possible for nurses with other commitments to work, there have been some experiments with other arrangements, for example based on the more traditional working pattern found outside nursing, sometimes referred to as the 9 to 5 pattern.

Different ways of organising nursing work have had a major impact on the organisation of the nurse's day. In many wards the system has moved from one of task assignment, whereby the nurse's day is decided by a series of tasks that the sister or nurse in charge allocates her to do, to one of far greater autonomy for the individual nurse, whereby the nurse's day revolves largely around the needs of her patients, and the nurse has to plan and set priorities.

Organising the nursing team and nursing care

A number of factors affect the way that a nursing team is organised on a ward, the main ones being the following, according to Matthews (1987):

- staffing levels;
- ratio of qualified nurses;
- ward design, for example Nightingale, race track, small rooms;
- patient turnover;
- type of patients nursed in the ward.

As mentioned before, the philosophy or beliefs held about nursing on the ward have an important bearing on the type of organisation chosen. There are two main ways of organising nursing – team nursing and primary nursing. Primary nursing is a complete system in itself, but two alternative approaches can be used in team nursing – allocation of jobs (task assignment) or allocation of patients (case assignment). These systems and sub-systems result in higher or lower degrees of personalisation, that is, the extent to which the nursing care is planned and provided on an individual patient basis. Vaughan and Pilmoor (1989) show how the different combinations of the main system with the sub-systems facilitate different degrees of personalisation of the service. Task allocation for a whole group of patients is the least personalised whereas primary nursing is the most highly personalised (see Fig. 3.4).

Fig. 3.4   The degree of personalistion found in different systems of nursing
             (Source: Vaughan and Pillmoor 1989)

Level of personalisation	*System combination*		
I N C R E A S I N G	Task allocation	to task teams	Task allocation to team members for whole patient group
	Patient allocation	to patient teams	Team allocation to team members for team/patient group only
P E R S O N A L I S A T I O N	Patient allocation	to patient teams	Patient allocation to individual team members — Total patient care while on duty
	Patient allocation	to primary nurse	Total patient care for entire need for nursing

In team nursing, the ward is divided into two or three teams, each with a team leader. The allocation of patients to teams is sometimes done on the basis of geography, e.g. Team 1 nurses all patients in Bays A and B, and Team 2, in Bays C and D, or Team 1 nurses patients on one side of a Nightingale-style ward and Team 2, the other side. Sometimes, patients are allocated to a team on the basis of their nursing dependency and an attempt is made to get a balance of low- and high-dependency patients in each team. On some wards the composition of each team remains relatively constant, at least for several weeks or even months; on others new teams are allocated at each shift and team leaders are appointed. The advantages of relatively permanent teams allocated to more or less the same group of patients is that continuity of care is facilitated and the nurses get to know their patients better; the disadvantages are that nurses do not necessarily get a range of experience (though that depends on the type of patients in each group) and personality conflicts may be exacerbated by the same nurse always caring for the same patients.

The role of the team leader is important. Matthews (1987) lists fourteen responsibilities of the team leader including: assignment of team members to their patients; participating herself in care of patients; planning care together with the nurse concerned; supervising and supporting team members; assessing the effectiveness of care; ensuring that students have opportunities to learn; keeping the ward sister informed of changes; and ensuring that the patient is well-informed about his care. In other words, the team leader needs to be able to assess, plan, implement and evaluate whilst attempting to to get the balance right between providing care herself and ensuring that others are providing high standard care. Some find this balance difficult to achieve since it entails all the skills of effective management.

There is a difference between allocation and delegation in team nursing. If a nurse has a number of patients simply allocated to her, she will need to refer back to the team leader or nurse in charge for advice and direction. If the team leader or nurse in charge has delegated the responsibility to other nurses, she then acts in a co-ordinating role, ensuring that the responsibility is exercised effectively. Before delegating, she needs to ask herself if the nurse:

- has the ability to give prescribed care with attention to detail and standards, with knowledge of patient needs, nursing and medical prescription;
- can attend to individual needs;
- has the skill and training necessary to perform the care.

In order to safeguard the delegation of responsibility, the nurse in charge should:

- talk with the nurse, checking her knowledge and skill, inviting her to ask what she needs to know;

- give the nurse sufficient relevant information;
- encourage the nurse to report on the patient's main problems and concerns;
- encourage the nurse to return for advice and guidance.

Primary nursing is a system that personalises care on a one-to-one basis, twenty-four hours a day, seven days a week, from admission to discharge. It has already been described in Chapter 2 and is again referred to in Chapters 5 and 8. The primary nurse is responsible for assessing the patient's nursing needs, planning care for each twenty-four-hour period, setting goals with the patient, providing care when on duty, evaluating its effectiveness, teaching patients and relatives, liaising with doctors and other health care workers, planning discharge and communicating effectively to ensure the continuity of care (Matthews 1987). This delegation of the responsibility for planning and delivery of nursing to the primary nurse affects the role of the nurse in charge. Vaughan and Pillmoor (1989) suggest that it allows the nurse in charge to concentrate on the following:

- clarification of the conceptual framework from which the practice of the ward arises;
- general mangement of the ward, including control of the ward budget;
- acting as clinical nurse consultant to other members of the nursing staff;
- developing expertise in a particular area of nursing in order to act as a specialist;
- responsibility for staff appraisal and development;
- research from a clinical base;
- the educational experience of students.

The role of the newly qualified nurse in management varies with the different models of nursing organisation. With the more traditional forms such as task allocation, the role of the nurse in charge is quite different from that described above for primary nursing. The nurse in charge of the ward will need to decide on the allocation of tasks to the whole patient group and will expect the team members to report back to her on completion of the tasks. She will act as the main liaison between nurses and doctors and with patients' relatives, since no other nurse has responsibility for individual patients. This makes being in charge quite an onerous task because the nurse in charge is expected to know so much and to respond to many questions from a variety of sources. Where there is individual patient assignment, enquiries can and should be directed to the nurse who has responsibility for the relevant patient; and, for example, it is more appropriate for that nurse to accompany a doctor's round when her group of patients is being discussed.

Skill mix

The nursing skill mix of a ward refers to the proportions of trained nurses, both registered and enrolled, and untrained staff including students (unless supernumerary) and auxiliaries and/or health care assistants. The skill mix of a ward depends on a number of factors including the following:

● the philosophy of care adopted by the ward;
● nature of the care required by patients and their 'dependency' on nursing care;
● hospital and health authority policies;
● the system for organising the nursing work;
● staff availability;
● nursing costs.

Sometimes, the actual skill mix of a ward is outside the control of the ward manager or nurse in charge because of external influences. However, it is possible for the ward manager to attempt to make out a rational case for the nurses they need, based on assessment of care needed, dependency studies and ward audits (see, for example, Binnie 1986 and Chalmers 1990). In the first example (Binnie 1986) the outcome in terms of skill mix was to opt for a higher proportion of registered nurses and a diminution of enrolled nurses and auxiliaries as a more cost-effective way of providing high-level nursing care (Pembrey 1989).

Achieving the most effective skill mix is increasingly being recognised as important, and is therefore an aspect of ward management that all nurses should be aware of. Further, the phasing out of the enrolled nurse training, the introduction of the health care assistant or support worker and the supernumerary status of students as a result of Project 2000 (see Chapter 8) will have major effects on the ward skill mix.

Budgeting and resource control

The newly registered nurse may have a lesser or greater involvement in ward finances and resources depending on the expectations of more senior nurses, particularly the ward sister, and the extent to which the responsibility for different aspects is devolved to different members of the ward team. Nevertheless, an understanding of how the budget is determined, and a greater awareness of costs and resource usage are important for all nurses.

With the implementation of the Griffith's management structure, the responsibility for budgeting within the NHS has been fully devolved to those managers who control resources. This includes the sister or nurse in charge of the ward, who, for the first time in many instances, becomes a budget holder, accountable for the use of the resources within her budget. Sisters are known as 'Facility Budget Holders', whereas departmental heads are 'Support Service Budget Holders', responsible for 'selling' the ward sister such services as catering and laundry. Clinicians or consultants are 'Clinical Budget Holders' who are charged by facility and department budget holders for services used by their patients.

Budget holders are allocated a certain amount of money following full discussion with the unit accountant. For ward sisters, the resources included in this budget will vary but will almost definitely include nursing manpower and possibly materials and equipment. Therefore, it is important for the nurse in charge to monitor the use of resources such as linen, disposables, dressings and stationery and to encourage the members of the nursing team to be economical in their use. One way that has been found very effective in raising cost-consciousness is to label items on the ward with price tags. This can be done by one or more of the ward nurses as a 'project' to inform the rest of the ward staff.

If the budget allows some degree of 'virement', that is, the movement of monies between different categories, this can be a great incentive for the better use of resources. So, for example, with some budgets, if money is saved on staffing it can be used to send one or more nurses on study days of their choice. The management of budgets and information about resources has been the focus of considerable change in the past few years. This is discussed further in Chaper 8.

While all the trained nurses should know about the supplies that are available and needed by the ward, it is better if one (or possibly two nurses) are solely responsible for the actual ordering of them. This allows familiarity with the ordering system, a more detailed knowledge of the ward stock requirements, a decreased tendency to overstock, more likelihood that deficiencies will be noted, and a greater attention to the budget implications. A system for filing copies of orders and for storing order books is important should there be queries about orders or a budget review.

Control of the physical environment

Ward management includes making sure that the environment is as conducive as possible for the well-being of patients and is safe for patients, visitors and staff. This includes factors such as ventilation, light, cleanliness, and control of noise as well as tidiness and aesthetics. Some of these aspects are outside the direct control of the ward manager; for example, the general cleanliness of the ward is largely the responsibility of the domestic team but any problems should be discussed first with the department concerned and then if necessary with the unit nurse manager. Cleanliness involving patient care equipment, such as mouth trays and suctioning apparatus, is the responsibility of the nurse and should be an automatic part of caring for the patient. Extra care should also be taken where there is a risk of cross-infection.

Control of noise, too, can in part be influenced by the nurse. Ill patients are often more sensitive to noise and its presence can interfere with their comfort and even recovery. Again, it is a useful 'project' for one or more nurses to identify the range of noise e.g. people talking loudly, equipment, radios and televisions, doors banging, squeaking trolleys and wheelchairs, and try to see what can be done to eliminate them. Sometimes nurses themselves are unaware of the noise they make. The new nurse to the ward should stand back from time to time and reflect on the amount of noise staff are making, for example talking with a colleague rather louder than is necessary at the nurses' station, particularly at night.

Looking at the aesthetics of the ward is something that all nurses can do. This can be enhanced in a variety of ways; for example by assisting patients to keep flowers and plants presentable, by the introduction of pictures and posters, by the use of colourful, non-institutional materials in curtaining if ward funds and hospital policies will allow this, and by the removal of clinical material from lockers and tables when no longer required.

Health and safety at work

Under the Health and Safety at Work Act 1974, every employer has a duty to ensure the health, safety and welfare at work of all his employees so far as is reasonably practical. In turn, every employee has a duty while at work to take reasonable care for the health and safety of himself and other persons who may be affected by his actions or omissions. Lifting and manoeuvring patients, the handling of toxic drugs, the movement and handling of large equipment and machinery related to patient care, the cleanliness of the environment and the safe handling of patients' food are just a few relevant examples (Rowden 1984).

Every nurse should be alert to a number of potential hazards on the ward such as spillages of both toxic chemicals and, indeed, more or less any fluid, equipment or furniture in a poor state of repair, and the careful disposal of waste and sharps in order to prevent accidents. Should an accident occur, however trivial, it must be reported in case of a complaint, a coroner's inquest or an insurance claim. If the accident involves a patient, visitor or nurse a special form should be completed by the nurse concerned, including the relevant details of the accident, the names, location and number of people involved, the cause (if known) of the accident, the nature of the injury, the equipment that was implicated, the action that was taken, the outcomes and, in the case of a patient, his physical and emotional state before and after. Names of witnesses are included where appropriate. It is important to record this information as soon after the event as possible, since the power of recall diminishes rapidly and it may be needed some months or even years after the incident.

Although the recording of the relevent information is the responsibility of the nurse or nurses involved, the nurse in charge at the time should also ensure that the correct procedures are implemented. This of course assumes that these are known; it is important, therefore, for even the most junior nurse to find out what to do in the event of an accident or incident.

Retrospective analysis of events related to accidents and incidents offers a learning opportunity and may prevent the situation reoccurring. Examples of accidents for discussion are: a patient receives incorrect medicines due to a faulty infusion pump; a patient falls when leaving her bedside. Examples of incidents are: the loss of a patient's valuables; a member of staff injures her back when lifting a patient.

The following questions can be asked of such an event:

- What was the event?
- What and who were involved?
- Could it have been avoided?
- What working practices should be changed to prevent the situation reoccurring?

Actively educating and increasing the awareness of the nursing team is a managerial function. Some methods for achieving this are as follows:

- Spend ten minutes analysing the situation as described.
- One staff nurse gives a short talk inviting nurses to draw up a list of safety hazards on the ward.
- Display policies describing hospital practices in prominent places, preferably at the location relevant to the policy, e.g. policies regarding the storage of patients' food should be placed in the kitchen; the sluice/dirty utility should have a waste disposal policy near the waste bins.
- Invite hospital safety representatives to discuss safety issues with the nursing team.

For further information on this topic, see Salvage and Rogers (1988).

Management of standards on the ward

The setting of standards in nursing care has already been discussed in Chapter 2 and is mentioned again in Chapter 8. The management of standards for the ward is, however, an important managerial function and one that has rightly received increasing prominence in recent years. Following the Government White Paper (DoH 1989), setting and monitoring standards is likely to become the norm for all wards eventually.

Standards for a ward should be based on achievable objectives and then incorporated into the unit profile. One useful way of setting standards for a ward is by the use of a quality circle. This has been described as a small group of 'volunteers working in the same area who meet regularly to identify, select and solve problems. The solution to the problem is then implemented and monitored to establish if the problem has been solved, (Sale 1990).

The essence of a circle is the voluntary participation of individuals who want to discuss and debate issues as peers and colleagues. It may be appropriate for the ward sister to lead the group, particularly initially, but if it is to achieve success, every member must have the opportunity to decide what they want to discuss and to contribute to the debate. Decisions should be the result of a consensus rather than the view of the leader; the leader's role is one of facilitation. The size of the group and the frequency of the meetings are also subjects for joint consideration. For guidance on how a quality circle works, see Robson (1984).

When standards have been set they will need to be monitored, and, importantly, reviewed in the light of experience and changing circumstances. A number of 'tools' have been developed to help assess the achievement of set standards, including the Phaneuf Nursing Audit (Phaneuf 1976), Monitor (Goldstone *et al.* 1983) and QUALPAC (Wandelt *et al.* 1974). Alternatively, some places have developed their own methods for auditing, which are specifically designed to meet their needs (see for example, Orr 1986 and Orr and Bryant 1990). A good deal has been written about standard setting and assessment and for more detail of the different approaches the reader is recommended to Pearson (1987), Kitson (1989) and Sale (1990).

Managing work in teams and with individual patients

Whether a system of team nursing or primary nursing is adopted, the newly registered nurse will need to manage a group of patients and provide care for individual patients.

Individual patient need assessment

The management of patient care starts with an assessment of the patient's needs, undertaken, if possible, in conjunction with the patient himself. If the nurse is in charge or is acting as a team leader, she is unlikely to undertake a detailed assessment herself, except of any patients that she herself is directly responsible for. As a manager – of the ward or team – she will need to ensure that a skilled assessment is performed by the nurses in her team, and that any students involved have the support of a trained member of staff. Her role will be a monitoring and co-ordinating one. She will probably undertake a brief assessment of the patients and assign the patients to the nurses if this has not already been done. This is a difficult skill to achieve for the relatively inexperienced nurse and the following points could be borne in mind:

- Is the allocation of patients to nurse usually done on a geographical basis?
- Has the patient been looked after by a particular nurse on previous shifts – continuity of care is often important?
- Does the group of patients assigned to one nurse give a reasonable spread of high-dependency and low-dependency patients?
- Does a particular patient require a specific nursing skill that only certain nurses on the ward have?

She then needs to set up a way of ensuring that the assessment has been properly carried out. This is usually best done by the individual nurses reporting back to the nurse in charge, or, alternatively, at a handover meeting where the relevant group of nurses passes on information about the patients they have cared for.

It is sometimes difficult for the relatively junior staff nurse to get the right balance between allowing other members of the team to get on with the work and getting feedback and information which enables monitoring to take place. Also, some sisters encourage more junior nurses to be in charge when they themselves are on duty, but acting as a team member rather than the ward leader. This can be daunting at first for the newly registered nurse who perhaps is more used to being led rather than herself leading. It works especially well, though, when the ward sister sees her role as supporting the more junior nurse whilst, at the same time, taking more of a back seat herself.

Clinical management

Once the nurse responsible for the patient has assessed his needs, the clinical management of the patient is planned. This involves *setting priorities* and *deciding on knowledge needed* and *action to be taken*. The team leader or ward manager may well be involved in this process, though possibly more as a consultant or colleague.

The priorities may be learnt by communicating with the patient (if this is possible) and the relatives, by observation and by questioning the nurse most recently caring for the patient. Priorities identified can cover the patient's capacities (what he can and cannot do); the patient's main anxieties and emotional state; the medical plan and the relationship to and role of family and friends. From this and other information, such as that gained from other members of the multidisciplinary team, the plan of management is drawn up. In developing the nursing plan, the nurse needs to take account of a number of factors including the clinical and social objectives. It is helpful in the management of the care of a patient to ascertain them and record them in the documentation for each patient. A social objective is a statement which enables the nurse to know the current social plan of each patient. If multidisciplinary meetings are held with social workers, physiotherapists, medical staff, and so on, the objective can be derived from this meeting.

The nurse in charge can use a discussion of the documentation as a means of finding out what care is planned for a patient and subsequently given. Though research has shown that detailed, regular recording is not always achieved, particularly in terms of the evaluation of care (Lathlean *et al.* 1986), and that some nurses view record keeping as an unnecessary intrusion on their time with patients, a written assessment, plan (including clinical and social objectives), description of the care given and evaluation of the outcome both helps the nurse to be systematic in her care for patients and the manager to offer support and guidance, as well as to ensure that the appropriate care is being given.

There has been a great deal written about managing patient care on an individualised basis, sometimes referred to as the nursing process. This uses the above-mentioned steps of assessing, planning, implementing and evaluating and lays importance on accurate and full recording. For additional information the reader is recommended to a succinct and practical overview of the steps to be taken given in the chapter entitled, 'Individualized patient care', in Matthews (1987). A more extensive but still practical coverage of the subject is to be found in the Open University Package, *A Systematic Approach to Nursing Care* (revised edition).

Discharging a patient

If primary nursing is practised it is the responsibility of each primary nurse to arrange for the discharge of her own patients. However, even with team nursing this is not always left to the nurse in charge so it is important for all nurses to be aware of the procedures.

Research has shown that whilst the need for assessment and planning to commence at the point of admission is stressed, too often plans are not considered until a decision to discharge has been made (Cass 1978). Roberts (1975) found little information relating to discharge in the medical records and none at all in the Kardex, and Skeet (1970) identified other shortcomings arising from nursing practice in connection with discharge, in particular the breakdown of communication about patients' needs that often occurs between colleagues, and poor transfer of information into the community. In a more recent research study of discharge planning in four geriatric wards, Waters (1987) concluded that whilst her findings tended to be more favourable than the previously mentioned two studies by Roberts and Skeet, discharge planning was not seen as a priority by ward nurses and doctors and that the present methods of communicating with patients in hospital need to be supplemented by written information. She further suggested that 'accurate, accessible and complete records are a prerequisite for effective discharge planning' (Waters 1987).

In a survey conducted by Vaughan and Taylor (1988) of patients discharged from hospital after surgery, one of the main findings was the need for more information prior to discharge, particularly on the rate and pattern of recovery, the 'do's' and 'dont's' to aid recovery, and the tiredness and potential loneliness. It was suggested that written advice would be especially helpful. It was further considered that there was a need for a named person to turn to for advice and support, and for help when first at home.

In order to plan effectively for discharge the nurse will need to know the following:

- What capacities does the patient have, i.e. what he can or cannot do?
- Where are his resources at home, e.g. if he is weak who will cook or shop?
- What learning will be necessary prior to discharge, e.g. taking medicines, appropriate diet, managing his oxygen?
- What does the patient feel about any adjustments that will be necessary in his lifestyle?

Matthews (1987) suggests that the steps to be taken when planning discharge are as follows:

- liaising with patient and doctor and arranging a suitable date;
- discussing discharge arrangements with the patient;
- liaising with patient's relatives or friends;
- liaising with other health care workers;
- arranging transport;
- arranging attendance at the outpatient department;
- arranging drugs, dressings, lotions required at home;
- arranging the doctor's letter for the patient's general practitioner;
- obtaining valuables, clothes and suitcases;
- providing medical certificates and completing benefit forms.

The information given to those involved in the subsequent care of the patient, e.g. the district nurse, should be as substantial as time and circumstances allow, and include details of the patient's capacities and the treatment he has already received.

The most important administrative activities need to be recorded. Fig. 3.5 illustrates a possible checklist which is straightforward and simple, but which has been used successfully on a medical ward for the discharge arrangements of patients (see also Skeet 1983).

A number of hospitals now have booklets or written information that the patient can take on discharge. One such booklet has been tested with surgical patients in Oxfordshire and preliminary evaluation seems to confirm its usefulness for the majority of patients receiving it. (See Vaughan 1988.)

Fig. 3.5   Example of a discharge checklist

SUPPORT SERVICES			
Prior to Admission		Needed	Arranged
	District Nurse Home Help Meals on Wheels Comm. Physio Comm. O.T. Area S.W. Others		
(P.T.O. to record details/addresses/tel. nos.			
TRANSFER/DISCHARGE PLAN			
Planned date: to:			
Patient advised:			
Relatives advised:			
Transport: Type: needed/arranged Escort: needed/arranged			
OPD:			
TTA'S:			
Other Information:			

Patients' rights

One of the key aspects of the nurses' role in managing the care of patients is to act as advocates and guardians of their rights. The accepted rights of patients are based on ethical principles. These are generally felt to be the following (Thompson *et al.* 1983; Fromer 1981):

● the right to know;
● the right to privacy;
● the right to treatment:
● the right to self-determination.

Patients have a right to be adequately informed of their condition, of plans for treatment and what these entail including possible adverse effects. It is the responsibility of health carers to ensure that information is adequate. This includes the terminally ill, who, it is now widely accepted, have a right to know the seriousness of their condition. Patients also have a right to privacy, and to confidentiality regarding their own personal details and illness history. Nurses have the responsibility to ensure that such confidentiality is maintained. Some difficulties arise in this area when respect for an individual's confidences and the wider public interest are in conflict. For example, in a situation where, during a confidential interview, a patient admits physically abusing a child, breaching the patient's rights is justified in the interests of the child and, depending on the circumstances, possibly other children that might be at risk.

Issues about breaking confidences are often difficult and their resolution may not be obvious. The UKCC Code of Professional Conduct (UKCC 1984) states that disclosure of confidential information without the consent of the individual is only allowed where required by law or where necessary in the public interest, and the advisory document which elaborates this point makes it clear that breaches of confidences should be exceptional (UKCC 1987). However, as Melia (1989) points out in a useful discussion of the topic, general principles are fine until the real situation is confronted. This tends to be far messier than 'theory' prepares us for, and therefore is often left to the professional and moral judgements of individuals in deciding what is best.

Patients also have the right to treatment and to self-determination, and therefore the right to refuse treatment if that is their wish. Closely bound up with these rights is the legal duty to gain informed consent from patients to any treatment or procedure. Informed consent implies not merely that a person has signed a consent form, but has been given clear and understandable information regarding the treatment or procedure, including its risks, benefits and alternatives, and that the individual understands this information. Coercion and pressure must not be placed upon the individual in order to gain his consent. The responsibility of gaining consent lies with the doctor or the person administering the treatment or procedure. Written consent must be gained for invasive procedures such as surgery; and for children and young people under the age of 16, consent is required from parents or guardian.

Breaches in obtaining true informed consent have resulted in the Department of Health publishing new guidelines and forms for obtaining consent from patients (DoH 1990). The instructions to patients on these forms spell out, in clear language, what consent means, and that they have a right to request a nurse or other individual to be present during the process of being given information and being asked to give their consent. Patients are also advised that they can refuse to be involved in the training of doctors or other health professionals without this affecting their care or treatment.

Written informed consent is also required for patients taking part in research as research subjects. It is the responsibility of the hospital ethical committee to ensure that patients' rights and safety are protected in research being undertaken on them, but it is also necessary for the individual researcher to adhere to ethical principles while undertaking research. Nurses need to be aware of any research involving patients in their care, and to request relevant research protocols which outline how the study is being conducted, how patients are selected for the study and how informed consent is gained, so that it is possible to scrutinise the studies themselves to ensure that patients' rights are being protected. Thus nurses have an important role to play in acting as guardians of patients' rights and safety in relation to research.

The rights of patients raises the question of the nurse's role as the patients' advocate. It is acknowledged that patients entering hospital are vulnerable; they are usually ill, dependent on a group of 'professional' people for their treatment and are often expected to play submissive 'sick role'. As such, even normally assertive and articulate individuals can find it difficult to ask for information or to be fully involved in decisions made about their treatment. The UKCC Code of Professional Conduct is clear about the nurse's role in this respect and states that 'each registered nurse . . . shall act always in such a way as to promote and safeguard the well being and interests of patient/clients [and] ensure that no action or omission on his/her part or within his/her sphere of influence is detrimental to the condition or safety of patients/clients'.

The nurse is usually the person in the health care team that the patient knows best and is likely thus to turn to for information, support and reassurance. Therefore the nurse must take this responsibility very seriously, by trying to see the situation through the eyes of the patient, and by defending and promoting the rights of the patient (Brower 1982). This may entail being a 'go-between' when other health care professionals appear to the patient to be unapproachable. Since the role of the advocate has been defined as 'to inform the client and then support him in whatever decision he makes' (Kohnke 1982, quoted in Webb 1987), it may also entail the nurse explaining to the patient possible alternative lines of treatment, so that he is fully aware of the implications before consent to treatment is given (Burnard and Chapman 1988).

Another aspect of the patient's rights is that of complaints. Patients who for some reason are dissatisfied with the service they receive may complain. This may range from the misplacement of an article of clothing to a much more serious complaint regarding the quality of their care, or perhaps even a criminal offence. Hospitals have complaints and grievance procedures which outline how such situations should be handled. More minor complaints can usually be resolved by discussing the problem. However, for other complaints patients and relatives should be advised of their rights to complain formally, and of the procedure for doing this.

Managing oneself

So far the emphasis has been on managing the ward and managing patient care. Indeed, management is often thought to apply to other people but managing oneself is important too, particularly at a time when many have difficulty in adjusting – the transition from student to staff nurse (Lathlean *et al.* 1986). A useful book that focuses on self-management and includes guidance on how to be more aware of oneself, as well as how to assert and support oneself, is that by Tschudin (1990).

For the newly registered nurse, a number of aspects are important, for example adjusting to the new role and to different people's expectations particularly medical staff and relatives, managing one's own time and the distinction between work and non-work, deciding on priorities, reviewing practice and performance, managing one's own stress and planning for the future.

Managing the transition

Most nurses will remember the feeling of pride experienced when going on to the ward for the first time as a staff nurse. Dale, on giving her thoughts as a newly qualified staff nurse, describes how, on her first day, she 'floated on to the ward' in her brand new uniform, preened herself in front of her colleagues 'like any fashion model' but was brought down to earth since 'the rest of the day was to prove less glamorous and [her] dignity far from intact' (Dale 1985). Chapters 1 and 2 both look at some of the factors that tend to make the transition problematic, but what can be done to ease it?

Some health authorities have realised the difficulties and have implemented staff development programmes for newly registered nurses (see, for example, Lathlean *et al.* 1986). These can range from a few days to schemes taking place over a much longer period up to eighteen months. The essence of many of the schemes is the provision of support and knowledge to nurses working in clinical areas. Sometimes participants stay in one clinical area for the whole of the programme; in other schemes there is rotation between two or three specialties to give different types of experience. Participants usually attend study days on topics relevant to the role of the staff nurse.

Some of the benefits of the schemes include the opportunity to get together with colleagues and to discuss problems and topics of mutual interest in an atmosphere that is supportive and non-judgemental, the chance to consolidate existing knowledge and skills and (normally) the ability to spend time with a 'facilitator' – someone who can assist in the learning process but who is not the direct manager of the nurse. Even if a health authority does not have a special programme, however, some of the features can be implemented in a more modest way. For example, the newly registered nurses can be 'attached' to a more senior or experienced nurse on the ward who then acts as a mentor, and opportunities can be made for groups of newly registered nurses to come together in a seminar or support group to discuss important issues. (This idea of a mentor for all newly registered nurses is being promoted by the UKCCs PREP project – see Chapter 9 for further details of this.)

There are a number of additional ways in which the newly registered nurse can develop her skills of management. For example, the nurse can:

- shadow a more senior nurse or ward sister and learn by role modelling;
- ask for feedback on performance of a managerial activity such as writing an off-duty rota, disciplining a member of staff or organising a patient's discharge;
- work out a plan of action with a colleague, put it into action and then discuss the results with a more senior nurse or group of nurses;
- identify 'critical incidents' (satisfying or worrying) that have occurred over a period of time, reflect on how she dealt with them and think through alternative strategies.

Time management

As Vaughan (1989b) suggests: 'It is very easy to fill one's day with things one likes doing, to the cost of things that are less enjoyable but nevertheless important.' In addition, there never seems to be enough time or it feels as though the time is misused. Binnie's (1988) study of the working lives of staff nurses illustrates this well. In a typical comment, one of the staff nurses said:

> We were really busy, we had twenty four patients in twenty beds. It was really horrible. And I didn't feel as if I had done anything, but I had always been doing something. But I hadn't done anything for the patients as such, I hadn't given anyone a bedpan or . . . .

Some nurses feel dissatisfied if they are not 'doing something directly' for the patient, such that a day spent in organising care, liaising with departments, answering the telephone, dealing with visitors, speaking to doctors and others on the ward feels like a day wasted. This is often remedied, however, by the system of primary nursing because the managerial and administrative jobs relating to a patient are undertaken by the patient's nurse, which is much more logical and meaningful for the nurse. Conversely, where administrative and managerial tasks are fragmented the following is common:

> You book all these social services for the patients, but you don't really know –
> I mean you book the district nurse, but you haven't actually done the dressing

yourself, which is a bit stupid . . . and then you tend to talk to people about the patient and you haven't actually given them a bedbath and you don't know *yourself* what they can do, it's only from the report . . . it feels hypocritical.

(Binnie 1988)

One important aspect of time management is setting priorities. Some find it helpful to mentally or actually divide the tasks into things that must be done because they are essential to life and those things that they want to achieve because they contribute to the quality of life (Vaughan 1989b). Making lists can be useful in order of priority or urgency of tasks. If the tendency is to be unrealistic in what can be done in a day this only leads to frustration; it is far more satisfying to be modest in estimating what can be achieved. Time also needs to be built into the day for teaching, communication and for reflection and relaxation.

Managing stress

It is ironic that, in a profession centred around caring for others and with an emphasis on helping others to cope with the stressful situation of being ill and in hospital, nurses are not always good at managing their own stress. The relatively high rates of smoking and suicide amongst nurses seem to be indicators of this. There is a much greater recognition now that nurses are at risk and literature abounds on how to cope and manage one's own stress. Chapter 6 discusses this subject much more fully. The reader is also referred to Whitehead (1989), who gives many practical ways in which nurses can 'take the strain' including the keeping of a diary to record stressful incidents.

Conclusion

It is impossible to separate out totally the activities of management and managing from the other aspects of the role of the staff nurse, such as providing clinical care and teaching. The necessity to assess, plan, implement and evaluate pervade the job whether the focus is the whole ward, the team, the individual or the nurse herself. The newly registered nurse may not consider herself as manager, but she certainly needs the skills of organising, leading, setting priorities, deploying resources, motivating and evaluating – the essence of management.

References

Binnie, A. (1986) Level 6 'Skill Mix' Project, Unpublished Discussion Paper, Oxfordshire Health Authority.

Binnie, A. (1988) The Working Lives of Staff Nurses: A Sociological Perspective, Unpublished MA Thesis, University of Warwick.

Brower, H. (1982) 'Advocacy: what it is', *Journal of Gerontological Nursing*, Vol. 8, (3), pp. 141–3.

Burnard, P. and Chapman, C. (1988) *Professional and Ethical Issues in Nursing*, Chichester: John Wiley.

Cass, S. (1978) 'The effects of the referral process on hospital in-patients', *Journal of Advanced Nursing*, Vol. 3, pp. 563–9.

Chalmers, J. (1990) 'Making resource management work', *The Professional Nurse*, Vol. 5, No. 4, pp. 178–80.

Dale, J. (1985) 'Thoughts of a newly qualified staff nurse', in Sykes, M. (1985) *Licensed to Practise*, Eastbourne: Baillière Tindall.

Department of Health (1989) *Working for Patients*, London: HMSO.

Department of Health (1990) *A Guide to Consent for Examination or Treatment*, NHS Management Executive Report HC (90) 22.

FitzGerald, M. (1989) 'A unit profile', in Vaughan, B. and Pillmoor, M. (eds.) (1989) *Managing Nursing Work*, London: Scutari Press.

Fretwell, J. (1982) *Ward Teaching and Learning*, London: Royal College of Nursing.

Fromer, M. J. (1981) *Ethical Issues in Health Care*, St Louis: C. V. Mosby.

Goldstone, L., Ball, J. A. and Collier, M. M. (1983) *MONITOR – An Index of the Quality of Nursing Care for Acute Medical and Surgical Wards*, Polytechnics Products Ltd, Newcastle Upon Tyne.

Handy, C. (1985) *Understanding Organizations*, Harmondsworth: Penguin.

Herzberg, F. (1966) *Work and the Nature of Man*, New York: World Publishing Company.

Humphries, A. (1987) *The Transition from Student to Staff Nurse*, Unpublished BSc Thesis, Leicester University.

Kitson, A. (1989) *Standards of Care: A Framework for Quality*, London: Royal College of Nursing.

Kohnke, M. (1982) 'Advocacy: what is it?' *Nursing and Health Care*, Vol. 3 (6), pp. 314–18.

Lathlean, J., Smith, G. and Bradley, S. (1986) *Post-Registration Development Schemes Evaluation*, Kings College, University of London.

Lippitt, R. and White, R. K. (1958) 'An experimental study of leadership and group life' in Maccoby, E. E., Newcombe, T. M. and Hartley, E. L. (eds.) *Readings in Social Psychology*, 3rd edn, New York: Holt.

Maslow, A. (1954) *Motivation and Personality*, New York: Harper.

Matthews, A. (1987) *In Charge of the Ward*, 2nd edn, Oxford: Blackwell Scientific Publications.

McGregor, D. (1960) *The Human Side of Enterprise,* New York: McGraw Hill.

Melia, K. (1989) *Everyday Nursing Ethics*, London: Macmillan Education Ltd.

Ogier, M. (1982) *An Ideal Sister?* London: Royal College of Nursing.

Open University Package P553 (1989) *A Systematic Approach to Nursing Care,* Revised Edition, Milton Keynes: Open University Press.

Orr, I. (1986) 'Nursing audit', *Senior Nurse*, Vol. 4, No. 2.

Orr, I. and Bryant, R. (1990) 'Development of an audit system', *Senior Nurse*, Vol. 10, No. 9, pp. 14–15.

Pearson, A. (ed.) (1987) *Nursing Quality Measurement*, Chichester: John Wiley.

Pembrey, S. (1989) 'The development of nursing practice: a new contribution', *Senior Nurse*, Vol. 9, no. 8, pp. 3–8.

Phaneuf, M. (1976) *The Nursing Audit*, New York: Appleton Century Crofts.

Roberts, I. (1975) *Discharge from Hospital*, London: Royal College of Nursing.

Robson, M. (1984) *Quality Circles – a Practical Guide*, London: Gower.

Rowden, R. (1984) *Managing Nursing*, Eastbourne: Baillière Tindall.

Sale, D. (1990) *Quality Assurance*, London: Macmillan Education Ltd.

Salvage, J. and Rogers, R. (1988) *Nurses at Risk: A Guide to Health and Safety at Work*, London: Heinemann Nursing.

Schein, E. H. (1965) *Organizational Psychology*, Englewood Cliffs, NJ: Prentice Hall.

Skeet, M. (1970) *Home from Hospital: A Study of the Home Care Needs of Recently Discharged Hospital Patients*, Dan Mason Nursing Research Committee.

Skeet, M. (1983) *Discharge Procedure – Practical Guidelines for Nurses*, London: Nursing Times Publication.

Smith, P. and Redfern, S. (1989) 'Educational experiences in hospital wards', in Wilson-Barnett, J. and Robinson, S. (eds.) *Directions in Nursing Research*, London: Scutari Press.

Thompson, I. E., Melia, K. M. and Boyd, K. M. (1983) *Nursing Ethics*, Edinburgh: Churchill Livingstone.

Tschudin, V. with Schober, J. (1990) *Managing Yourself*, London: Macmillan.

United Kingdom Central Council for Nursing Midwifery and Health Visiting (1984) *Code of Professional Conduct for the Nurse, Midwife and Health Visitor*, 2nd edn., London: UKCC.

United Kingdom Central Council for Nursing Midwifery and Health Visiting (1987) *Confidentiality: An Elaboration of Clause 9 of the Second Edition of the UKCC's Code of Professional Conduct for the Nurse, Midwife and Health Visitor*, London: UKCC.

Vaughan, B. (1980) *The Newly Qualified Staff Nurse – Factors Affecting Transition*, Unpublished MSc Thesis, University of Manchester.

Vaughan, B. (1988) 'Discharge following surgery', *Nursing Times*, Vol. 84, No. 15, pp. 32–3.

Vaughan, B. and Taylor, K. (1988) 'Discharge procedures. Homeward bound', *Nursing Times*, Vol. 84, No. 15, pp. 28–31.

Vaughan, B. (1989a) 'Dilemmas in practice', in Vaughan, B. and Pillmoor, M. (eds.) *Managing Nursing Work*, London: Scutari Press.

Vaughan, B. (1989b) 'Managing time', in Vaughan, B. and Pillmoor, M. (eds.) (1989) *Managing Nursing Work*, London: Scutari Press.

Vaughan, B. and Pillmoor, M. (eds.) (1989) *Managing Nursing Work*, London: Scutari Press.

Wandelt, M. A. and Agar, J. (1974) *Quality Patient Care Scale, Qualpacs*, New York: Appleton Century Crofts.

Waters, K. (1987) 'Discharge planning: an exploratory study of the process of discharge planning on geriatric wards', *Journal of Advanced Nursing*, Vol. 12, pp. 71–83.

Webb, C. (1987) 'The nurse advocate', *Nursing Times*, Vol. 83 (34), pp. 33–5.

Whitehead, L. (1989) 'Taking the strain', in Vaughan, B. and Pillmoor, M. (eds.) *Managing Nursing Work*, London: Scutari Press.

Further Reading

Dodwell, M. and Lathlean, J. (1989) *Management and Professional Development for Nurses*, London: Harper and Row.

Marson, S., Hartlebury, M., Johnstone, R. and Scammell, B. (1990) *Managing People*, London: Macmillan.

Matthews, A. (1987) *In Charge of the Ward*, 2nd edn., Oxford: Blackwell Scientific Publications.

Rowden, R. (1984) *Managing Nursing*, Eastbourne: Baillière Tindall.

Tschudin, V. (1986) *Ethics in Nursing; The Caring Relationship*, London: Heinemann Nursing.

Vaughan, B. and Pillmoor, M. (eds.) (1989) *Managing Nursing Work*, London: Scutari Press.

4 Communication

CAROLINE SHULDHAM

Introduction

There is an increasing awareness of the central role that communication plays in nursing practice. It is after all a fundamental aspect of human relationships and has been identified as one of the activities of living (Roper *et al.* 1980). Nurses become familiar with communication both as a result of professional preparation as well as life experiences. Nevertheless, communication can present difficulties for the newly registered nurse. She has to make decisions about many things including how to ration time and attention fairly between individual patients (Melia 1987) and may feel guilty if seen talking to patients and relatives (Darbyshire 1987). In common with the sister (Runciman 1983) she has to communicate with a wide range of people and may have limited experience of doing so (see Fig. 4.1).

Often, for the first time, it is not possible to refer difficult questions or uncomfortable situations to someone else. As a professional the nurse also has to articulate her opinions, for example on a consultant's ward round, and may have to speak at multidisciplinary team meetings. In such situations the nurse's feelings of competence may be threatened and she may fear losing face. Yet as the nurse in charge she may have to continue to manage the ward, delegate work to others and act as mentor to student nurses. The newly registered nurse may also have to discuss with patients and their relatives many issues concerning diagnosis, progress and prognosis, and cope with the ensuing emotions. These examples highlight some of the problematic situations that the newly registered nurse may encounter.

In the light of this complex nature of communication, therefore, it is perhaps not surprising to find that many of the complaints received concerning health care relate to communication. Footitt (1981) cites the example of one health district where a review of one hundred complaints from patients regarding their care revealed that 25 per cent were due to a primary breakdown in communication. Furthermore, 50 per cent of the remainder had a communi-

Fig. 4.1   The range of communication (Adapted from Runciman 1983)

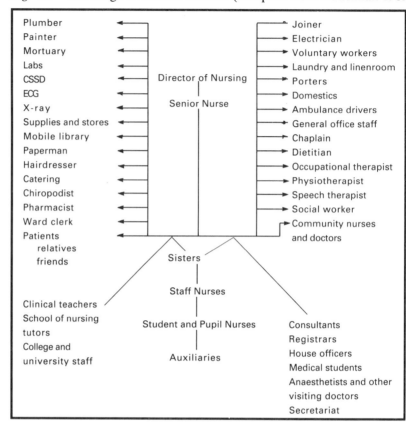

cation fault which was secondary to the main body of the complaint. Walton (1986) in her examination of the Health Service Ombudsman's reports groups the failures in communication which concern nurses under the following headings:

- failure to give relatives adequate or timely information;
- failure to summon (prompt) medical attention or to facilitate meetings between relatives and medical staff;
- failure to offer waiting patients or relatives reassurrance or explanations for delays;
- failures in communication between hospital and community care staff;
- unsympathetic staff attitudes;
- failure to keep proper records.

The nature of communication

Bridge and Macleod Clark (1981) suggest that communication means many different things to different people. One of the common notions among nurses seems to be that communication is concerned only with the giving of information, particularly to patients. However, as Fritz *et al.* (1984) point out it involves much more than this. They state that communication is a complex, intentional or unintentional process that includes a person formulating thoughts into a stimulus, transmitting that stimulus and receiving a response to that stimulus. One of the most important aspects of such a definition for nurses is the recognition that communication is a two-way process. Were it only one way then there would be no opportunity for feedback to check understanding (Bradley and Eidenberg 1982).

Fritz *et al.* (1984) remind the reader that communication may be unintentional. To take that idea further is to suggest that a person may be unaware of what is being communicated and may communicate something that had not been intended. It also means that the same thing said or done in respect of different people will have variable results. After all, communication is concerned with interaction between individuals. It is therefore subject to all the influences that individuals bring to any situation. Hargie and Marshall (1986) illustrate some of these in their model of interpersonal communication. These include the recognition that social interaction involves other people and that feelings and emotions are important. Hargie and Marshall (1986) also draw attention to the influence of perception, that is, the person's perception of what he or she is saying, of its effect on others and his or her perception of the responses of others.

This notion of perception is relevant to nursing. It can be tempting to think that if a person has been told something once then he will know, understand and remember it. In reality this is not the case and perhaps never more so than when a person is sick, under stress in unfamiliar surroundings and being given information which he does not wish to accept. The message may then be misunderstood or the response to it be misinterpreted. An example of this occurred when a nurse told a woman that her husband was dying. During repeated conversations with staff this fact was reiterated. However, when the man died his wife turned to the nurse saying: 'No-one told me he was going to die'. Her perception of the information and the nurse's were at variance.

The popular/unpopular patient

Factors other than perception influence communication. Hargie and Marshall (1986) argue that personal characteristics such as age, sex and appearance and situational factors, for example, roles and cultural background, are important influential elements in the communication process. These are of significance in nursing as there is evidence to suggest that nurses prefer some patients to others and evaluate them more favourably (Kelly and May 1982; Marshall 1985).

Many factors about patients have been found to influence their popularity including the nature of the judgements made by staff concerning patients (Kelly and May 1982).

Stockwell (1972) in her study *The Unpopular Patient* tested the hypotheses that there are some patients whom nurses enjoy caring for and who are more popular than others with nursing staff, and observable and measurable differences in the nursing care given to popular and unpopular patients. To do this she used a combination of rating and ranking techniques, a case study to compare wards, observation, and assessment of popular and unpopular patients, followed by semi-structured interviews with nurses. From this the patients whom nurses enjoy caring for and those who were least popular were identified as in Fig. 4.2.

Fig. 4.2   The popular and unpopular patient

The popular patient:
- was able to communicate readily with the nurses;
- knew the nurses' names;
- was able to joke and laugh with the nurses;
- co-operated in being helped to get well and expressed determination to do so.

The unpopular patient:
- grumbled and complained;
- communicated lack of enjoyment at being in hospital;
- implied they were suffering more than was believed by the nurses;
- suffered from conditions the nurses felt could be better cared for in other wards or specialised hospitals.

Further attempts have been made to elucidate this question of popularity. Marshall (1985) described a small study into the reactions of thirty-five patients and eighteen staff in a psychiatric setting. He found that staff viewed patients more favourably if they:

- had been in hospital for more than three months;
- had no previous psychiatric history;
- came from the indigenous population rather than from an ethnic minority;
- were not confined to the hospital grounds.

Work by Roberts (1984) in Australia has also provided information on the nature of popular and unpopular patients. Roberts used a questionnaire to survey 150 second and third year student nurses and asked them to rate patients' types according to how popular the nurses felt them to be. Fig. 4.3 shows the rank order found for the most unpopular patients.

Fig. 4.3   Rank order of unpopular patients (Source: Roberts 1984)

The most unpopular patients were found to be those who:
1. belong to the medical or nursing profession;
2. had been admitted because of intentional self-poisoning ('overdoses');
3. had been diagnosed as or suspected of having a drinking problem;
4. speak little or no English;
5. had been diagnosed as or suspected of being addicted to drugs (other than alcohol);
6. had been diagnosed as or suspected of having a psychiatric illness;
7. had been in hospital continuously for more than 3 months (approximately);
8. were relatives of terminally ill patients;
9. were aboriginal in origin;
10. asked a lot of questions about their treatment or investigations;
11. were terminally ill.

Using open-ended questions Roberts (1984) was also able to determine the patients that his sample of student nurses most liked and disliked caring for (see Fig. 4.4). Roberts (1984) concluded that the 'ideal' patient had a clearly defined, visible disability, was uncritical, submissive and appreciative of the care given.

Verbal/non-verbal communication

Nurses communicate to patients through verbal and non-verbal tactics. The verbal aspect of communication is the language of facts and things, the means by which people solve problems and apply logic. It is the language that can be written down. Non-verbal communication, on the other hand, is normally used to support verbal aspects, the signals being used to convey emotions and interpersonal attitudes (Argyle 1969). Argyle describes these visual and tactile stimuli as:

- bodily contact;
  hitting another person, showing aggression,
  stroking and the like which displays a nurturant behaviour,
  giving greetings or farewell, for example by shaking hands,
  holding another person to provide communication and companionship,
  guiding movements such as helping an elderly person to sit down;
- proximity;

Fig. 4.4 Most liked and disliked patients

Patients the nurses especially liked caring for   (the top ten)
1. Miscellaneous surgical patients
2. Miscellaneous patients 'interesting to nurse'
3. Cheerful patients with a sense of humour
   Elderly patients who are not senile
   Grateful appreciative patients
4. Children
5. Patients who help themselves
   Very sick patients – 'acute patients'
6. Uncomplaining patients
7. Terminally ill patients
8. Co-operative patients
9. Male patients
10. Patients who are genuinely ill

Patients the nurses especially disliked caring for
1. Patients who criticise the nurses or hospital
2. Demanding, selfish patients
3. Patients who do not help themselves when able to
4. Psycho-social problems
5. Lack of appreciation 'treated like a handmaiden'
6. Confused geriatrics
7. Stroke victims (CVAs)
8. Patients who ignore medical advice or treatment
   Patients who treat hospital like an hotel
9. Aggressive patients
10. Chronic patients

- posture;
- physical appearance;
- facial expression and gestures;
- direction of gaze.

Nurses use these aspects of non-verbal communication both during their interactions with peers and colleagues and when caring for patients. Some of the usual conventions may then be broken, for example in relation to proximity. Generally, the proximity between people should take account of an individual's personal space and is defined by the type of relationship between people. Nursing often necessitates contact between patient and nurse which is within the intimate/personal ranges, a degree of proximity only usually found between those well known to each other. The nurse has therefore to be sensitive to the individual's feelings about such contact and, as described later, may be able to capitalise on this and use touch in a therapeutic manner.

Physical appearance as a form of non-verbal communication is also important. It includes body type and personal adornment. Nurses usually wear a uniform and through that may convey messages of competence, authority and the like. In contrast, patients in hospital often have to give up their clothes, wear night attire and have jewellery removed. This may confirm in a person's mind his position as a sick person, may influence behaviour and may also reduce feelings of independence and self-worth. Jewellery in particular may serve as a comfort and reminder of normality. This aspect was illustrated by Edwards and Brilhart (1981) who cite the case of a young girl with leukaemia who, when in hospital, had to take off a gold chain and butterfly she always wore. She is quoted as saying 'I hate that, for it symbolises both love and hope in me', the implication being that nurses should consider all aspects of communication, even those that are not immediately obvious.

Communication skills

Effective communication therefore presupposes that the nurse utilises a range of skills. These are identified in Fig. 4.5.

Fig.4.5 Communications skills (Source: Macleod Clark 1984)

Observing and listening	to verbal and non-verbal cues
Reinforcing and encouraging patients to communicate	by: attending acknowledging praising supporting mirroring and reflecting
Questioning	open questions closed questions exploratory questions
Responding	to direct questions to indirect questions to statements and cues
Giving information	at appropriate time at approprite level in appropriate form

In contrast Tomlinson and Williams (1985) focus on:

- active listening;
- questioning;
- responding, encouraging and reinforcing;
- giving information;
- opening and closing conversations.

From this it can be seen that there are common elements, e.g. questioning and listening. Questioning in particular has received much attention, with nurses generally aware of the difference between closed and open questions such as 'Are you feeling all right today?' in contrast to 'how are you feeling today?' This first leading type of question is used to elicit structured, constricted information whereas the second 'open' question should elicit unstructured detail that should reflect the person's true state more accurately. Macleod Clark (1984) analysed the content of nurse–patient conversations on surgical wards, and found that nurses tended to use closed and leading questions and often failed to adopt exploratory or prompting questions to find information and direct the interaction. Words alone do not determine response.

Argyle (1969) recognises this by highlighting non-verbal aspects of speech; timing; emotional tone; speech errors and accent; the type of utterance; and, finally, structure. Importantly the nurse also has to listen, and demonstrate that by maintaining eye contact. Although this may sound obvious MacLeod Clark (1984) actually found that nurses did not always listen to the response to their questions and often did not use tactics such as mirroring and reflecting in order to encourage patients to communicate.

Patients then asked nurses relatively few questions. Instead they often employed indirect or implied questions or used a statement that required an answer. Nurses dealt with these by either:

- giving the appropriate information;
- being vague and avoiding the issue;
- completely ignoring the question.

This final tactic was used only occasionally. However, as Fritz et al. (1984) point out, 'to refuse to respond is to deny the existence of the other person'. It reflects a disconfirming approach (Heineken and Roberts 1983). In their work on confirming/disconfirming responses Heineken and Roberts (1983) state that to use a confirming response is to make the patient feel endorsed, acknowledged and accepted (see Table 4.1). This requires that the nurse is flexible, has an individual approach and does not adopt the tendency to use stock phrases (Fritz et al. 1984).

Different words may be used as well as variable types of responses. These can be classified as follows:

Table 4.1 Confirming/disconfirming tactics

Confirming	Disconfirming
Directly respond to the person's statements	Making irrelevant comments
Nod one's head	Responding ambiguously
Ask questions related to the same problems	Interrupting
Show verbal and non-verbal interest and awareness of what is being said	Keeping silent when a response is indicated
Express agreement, disagreement or neutrality	Failing to acknowledge an individual's communication
Expand or elaborate on content	Using impersonal language
Express feelings about the content	Introducing a different, unrelated topic
Repeat or request clarification of what the other says	Shifting the focus to a peripheral subject
	Avoiding or shifting eye contact
	Turning away from the speaker
	Tapping feet or fingers

Source: Heineken and Roberts 1983

- probing: to find out more information;
- interpretive: to gain understanding;
- evaluative: making a judgement;
- reflecting: re-stating what has been said;
- confronting: challenging in a non-aggressive fashion.

Interestingly, silence can be used as a probe rather than being viewed as uncomfortable (Fritz *et al.* 1984) and consequently avoided. This is the case whether talking to a person face to face or on the telephone. Similar tactics are used in both situations. However, when actually facing a person there is the added advantage of reading his non-verbal cues. Perhaps the most important aspect is that when communicating with patients, relatives, peers or colleagues it is essential that the nurse learns to accept the person as he is and to communicate this attitude to him. In so doing, the nurse communicates that she values the person who is at all times a human being, a member of a social group as well as an individual, and indicates by her manner that the patient/client may seek help or advice. Throughout the process the nurse has to be non-judgemental. Indeed, Lay (1979) argues that until nurses participate in non-judgemental listening, then it will never be possible to facilitate active participation in health care.

Communicating with patients and their relatives

Responding to difficult questions

Many nurses worry that if they explore how a patient feels about an illness they may be faced with difficult questions or strong and uncomfortable emotions such as anger, despair or grief (Maguire 1985). Indeed, Macleod Clark (1984) found that less than 1 per cent of nurse–patient conversations focused on patients' emotions and feelings. This may precipitate the situation reported by Maguire (1985) wherein social and psychological problems are unrecognised in up to 80 per cent of physically ill patients.

Ashworth's (1980) study illustrates some of the potential difficulties. She examined communication between nurses and patients in Intensive Care Units where the patient's normal mode of communication was impaired by oro-tracheal, naso-tracheal or tracheostomy tube which prevents audible speech. Observation was carried out in four Intensive Care Units and 112 staff and 22 patients were interviewed. Her findings suggest that many Intensive Care nurses do care about their patients as human beings. However, their approach to maintaining appropriate communication with each patient according to need was much less professional than other aspects of their care. The implication is that nurses need to plan care in order that essential communication needs are met.

This individual planning is important for all patients but particularly for those with communication difficulties, when information is likely to be misinterpreted, and in situations where bad news may be given. One of the most difficult problems faced by the newly registered nurse is whether and how much to tell dying patients about their illness, and yet rules about discussing issues such as diagnosis are not really useful (Maguire 1985). Even where the doctor feels the patient should not be told something and the nurses disagree, no hard and fast rules can be applied. Rather, information should be selected for each individual person. Knight and Field (1981) suggest that in reality communication between staff and patients is routinised and mainly restricted to technical matters. They found that this approach affected communication by:

● ensuring consistency in the sort of information which a patient or patients with similar conditions received;
● absolving doctors from having to take decisions in individual cases;
● ensuring that staff did not come into conflict over what patients should be told.

Despite these constraints patients do become suspicious about their diagnosis, but, deprived of the opportunity to discuss their problems openly, they are unable to have their opinions confirmed. Knight and Field (1981) studied thirteen terminally ill patients and found only five who were completely unaware of their condition despite the 'closed awareness' that operated. Patients had to seek out cues from symptoms, treatment, physical deterioration and the like. They also:

● paid special attention to the conversations around them, especially during ward rounds;
● directly questioned staff which although it might not lead to answers could reveal clues;

● used indirect questions to 'set traps' for staff.

One of the reasons why nurses may avoid discussing sensitive matters is that they fear the emotional outburst that may ensue, for example the patient or his family may cry. Authier *et al.* (1979) provide advice on coping with people who cry for a reason such as loss or disability:

● Do *not* discount the person's feelings by giving premature reassurance such as 'OK don't worry about it, everything will work out'.
● Desensitise yourself from it.
● Facilitate the patient experiencing the hurt by helping him to express his emotions and ventilate his feelings.
● Express support, reassurance and encouragement, pointing out his strengths and assets.

Finally, it is important to show empathy, to communicate an awareness or understanding of what the other person is experiencing. Empathy is orientated towards the feelings and can be demonstrated in several ways. Firstly, the nurse may reflect back what the person says. Through this the nurse may help the person feel he has the opportunity to explore and the permission to express feelings. Secondly, the nurse may then also use open-feeling-orientated questions. Thirdly, self-disclosure may help reduce the emotional distance between the two parties. Finally, Authier *et al.* (1979) suggest that the nurse may confront the patient. This must be differentiated from anger. Confrontation is used to get at the truth of a situation, e.g. 'you tell me you are fine but you look as if you have been crying', where verbal and non-verbal cues are at variance. The nurse must approach the patient with warmth, sincerity, respect and caring, for, as Lay (1979) points out, 'being professional all too frequently has meant delivery of services from behind a cool and distant professional image. Growing evidence suggests that an impersonal stance is counterproductive in health care'.

Talking to dying or bereaved people

Several issues concerning communication with dying patients have already been raised. There is no one right person to tell patients about their future (West and Kirkham 1983) and, fearing the emotional outburst, most people would choose to discuss issues concerned with diagnosis, prognosis and death face-to-face rather than over the telephone. Health professionals and patients may nevertheless avoid the issue. Hinton (1974) writes that doctors think patients do not wish to raise the subject of dying except to gain reassurance and that the truth is likely to be hurtful. In reality, he argues, denial of mortality prevents the person having the opportunity to question or discuss his illness, can make him feel isolated, and denies him the chance to order his family and business affairs and to find spiritual peace.

Obviously people have differing requirements and therefore an individual approach should be selected:

- Some people only wish to know a little about their illness and 'clearly an abrupt statement to every patient with incurable disease that he is going to die is likely to do more harm than good' (Hinton 1974).
- If the dying person indicates openly that he does not want to know, if he shows by his manner or by his talk that he does not wish to regard his illness as fatal it would be uncharitable to force the truth on him.
- When a loaded question is put it is often better not to answer the dying person's question straight away. Use reflection or probing to find out what is on his mind. Listen sympathetically.
- Allow the person to speak of his suspicions or knowledge of the outcome.
- If it is unclear whether a sick person wants to know the whole truth, give gentle hints and see where it leads.
- Allow awareness of the outcome to grow.
- Resolve conflicting opinions within the multidisciplinary team; establish common ground and find out what the patient knows (Hinton 1974).

West and Kirkham (1983), doctors at St Christopher's Hospice, studied 591 patients with malignant disease to determine their insight into their diagnosis. In conclusion they wrote: 'If we do not tell our patients the truth, perhaps without necessarily being asked, our patients may later ask *why* they have not been told . . ., one patient asked . . ., in a tone of disbelief, "Do you mean to say that my family and the nurses all know that I had cancer and I didn't? They must have been laughing their bloody heads off." '

Talking with the relatives

Relatives may be given information that is different from that told to the patient. This creates the risk that conflict, lack of trust and secrecy occur within the family. It can also mean that the patient lacks allies (Knight and Field 1981) or friends at a time when they are most needed. The DHSS circular *Patients Dying in Hospital* (1984) states that medical staff should take utmost care to ensure that relatives and friends are fully aware of the prognosis of a patient's illness and whether there is the possibility of sudden death. Nurses should provide full support to patients and their families and ensure that relatives are aware of any changes in a patient's condition that necessitates them being present at the hospital.

Support to relatives can be provided in the following ways (Hacking 1981):

- by listening to both the relatives and patient in order to help each towards an understanding of the others' feelings and the state of their present knowledge;
- seeing the relatives separately from the patient when appropriate;
- reassuring them that if they show their feelings or talk about the illness, the patient will probably be able to cope with it;
- encouraging discussion between the relatives and the patient about their mutual problems;
- being available, and present when needed;
- providing time to sit quietly with the relatives;
- giving clear instructions.

Providing reassurance

Reassurance is a term often used by nurses to describe an aspect of their communication with patients and their families. The meaning, however, can be imprecise. Reassurance is a nursing interpersonal skill used to restore a person's confidence in himself and in his treatment situation, i.e. confidence lost through fear of either the known or the unknown (French 1979). A common misconception is that reassurance is provided by helping the person avoid anxiety-provoking information. False reassurance is then given using such clichés as 'you'll be fine' and 'it will work out', whereas when a topic, problem or major concern emerges, talking it through to its conclusion will generally provide tangible, productive results (Shields 1984).

French (1979) provides clear guidelines for the nurse seeking to provide reassurance. When the patient fears the unknown:

1. Explain what is happening or going to happen. (This is not synonymous with reassurance but is only one aspect of it.)
2. Familiarise the person with an unfamiliar situation, e.g. on admission show the patient around the ward.
3. Introduce a familiar element into unfamiliar situations, e.g. a known person may accompany a patient to theatre.
4. Use touch.
5. Consider proximity: the physical presence of the nurse can be reassuring.
6. Convey emotional stability using non-verbal communication.
7. Counsel the patient and help him to use his own skills to overcome his fears.

When the person fears the known:

1. Clarify the facts to put their knowledge of the situation into the correct perspective.

Fig. 4.6 Communicating with confused or delirious patients (Source: Trockman 1978)

- Help restore the patient's ability to perceive the environment correctly by checking on the need for glasses, hearing aid or interpreter.
- Position the patient appropriately, i.e. if he is deaf in one ear approach from the functioning side.
- Use all senses, e.g. visual and auditory but do not either overload or deprive the patient.
- Bring in familiar objects.
- Approach the patient face-to-face and at the same level.
- Address the person by name.
- Use simple, short, direct statements.
- Provide aids such as paper and pencil where necessary.
- Explain to the patient what you are doing when providing care.
- Orientate him in time and place and use familiar reference points such as his occupation, family status, hobbies and the like.
- Remind the patient of what he can do.
- Repeat as often as required.
- Remain good natured and unflustered.

Fig. 4.7 Communicating with the manipulative patient (Source: McMorrow 1981)

McMorrow (1981) suggests that 'if when caring for a patient who is manipulative and abusive you begin to feel angry, depressed or confused, the patient is manipulating'.

- All staff should be both firm and consistent.
- Encourage the person to express his feelings.
- If he refuses to recognise the inappropriateness of his behaviour, refuse to play the game.

2. Enable the person to verbalise and ventilate his fears.
3. Where appropriate, use diversional tactics, e.g. conversation (French 1979).

Patients with special problems and needs

Certain patients have very particular problems in relation to communication which require the nurse to capitalise on all her communication skills. Some examples are outlined in Figs. 4.6, 4.7, 4.8 and 4.9, with suggested approaches to help facilitate effective communication with such people as those who are confused or delirious, manipulative, deaf or unconscious.

Fig. 4.8 Communicating with a patient who is unconscious (Source: Shuldham 1984)

- Capitalise on the senses thought to be intact: hearing, touch and sometimes sight.
- Use touch, sight, physical presence and smell to supplement verbal communication.
- Find out what the patient likes to be called and use that name.
- Introduce yourself to the patient.
- Talk to him as an adult and give him the sort of communication that will play a supportive role.
- Use clear, slow speech with normal phrasing and rhythm.
- Avoid jargon especially as the patient cannot ask for clarification.
- Be honest; bring the outside world to the patient.

Fig. 4.9 Communicating with a deaf person (Source: Beanlands and MacKay 1981)

- Use sign language and find someone accomplished in this e.g. a member of the famiy.
- Utilise relevant audiovisual material.
- When speaking to the person: do not face the light source
    stand 2–6 feet away
    do not speak when trying to carry out a task
    speak slowly, distinctly with good articulation
    stress key words
    use everyday words not technical terms or jargon
- Write important points down.
- Get the patient to demonstrate that he understands (do not rely on his smile!).
- Encourage the deaf person to use his voice.
- Maximise any residual hearing, e.g. with a hearing aid.
- Give written instructions that are simple, clear and concise.

Communicating with the multidisciplinary team

Attention has already been drawn to the fact that the nurse has to communicate with a range of people. As a qualified person she has to collaborate with others as a professional. The newly registered nurse can feel intimidated by groups or individuals, e.g. by doctors, in particular consultants, or by other participants in multidisciplinary team meetings. In these situations there is a need to be well prepared and knowledgeable, always to know the answer, to have instant recall and to be able to articulate opinions. The nurse needs to speak up for her rights and beliefs and to use her initiative. At the same time, however, the nurse may feel shy, lack confidence and be fearful of losing face by being made to look a fool. In these circumstances many experience apprehension or anxiety which can make the whole situation worse. Rather than focusing on her feelings it is vital that the nurse focus her attention on what others are doing or saying. This goes some way towards developing an assertive approach, one wherein the nurse speaks up and stands up for her own rights without infringing on the rights of others (Edwards and Brilhart 1981).

In her work on 'Stress and self awareness' Bond (1986) describes four approaches namely: assertive, aggressive, manipulative and submissive. These latter three, she argues, are non-assertive approaches. They can promote stress in the nurse because of a lack of respect from other people, failing to have one's needs met and from feeling bad about oneself. If nurses were more assertive, on the other hand, this would lead to less stress and a realistic degree of self-confidence. An assertive approach is one where the person:

● decides for himself and allows and enables others to decide for themselves;
● makes statements which are positive and to the point;
● uses the first person (I want, I think) thereby speaking for themselves;
● adopts assertive body language:

> Posture is relaxed, well balanced, upright, facing the other person, calm and relatively still. Gestures are open and relaxed and related to the points being made, otherwise the hands are relatively still. Eye contact is direct but relaxed, and at the same eye level whenever possible. Facial expression is relaxed, firm, open and pleasant without inappropriate smiles. Distance from the other person is at an average, comfortable proximity. The voice is relaxed and relatively low pitched, with a firm but gentle tone, enough volume to be heard clearly.
>
> (Bond 1986)

Obviously the non-verbal aspects of communication need to be considered alongside the verbal response. As Edwards and Brilhart (1981) suggest, it is imperative to be precise, avoid jargon and the sort of 'double speak' used to give the impression of having communicated. Bond (1986) also draws attention to the need to be precise but, in addition, recommends the following:

● working out what is wanted;
● giving a clear concise statement which expresses what is wanted with a relevant strength of feeling;
● attracting the person's attention and making sure that is assured before proceeding;

- being persistent by sticking to the request, or by fielding the response, i.e. listening carefully, responding to a question or summarising and repeating the statement;
- saying 'No' when that is what is meant.

Throughout it should be remembered that an assertive approach acknowledges not only the rights of the person making the statement, or request, or voicing an opinion, but also gives equal consideration to the rights of the other individual. This being the case the other person always has the right to decide for himself, to agree or disagree, to make mistakes and to change his mind.

Factors important to communication at ward level

There are many aspects of the ward climate that enhance communication within the multidisciplinary team and facilitate the use of the tactics outlined above. In the main these characteristics are inherent in a democratic style of ward management. Some influential factors are the following:

- The relationship between staff is that of professional associates, i.e. collegiate.
- Team members co-operate with each other to work together towards a common goal.
- The sister-in-charge makes opportunities for the nurses to communicate with her regularly.
- Each person has the freedom to express opinions.
- Staff listen to each other. There is a degree of goodwill and trust.
- Information is disseminated and explained.
- There is consultation before decisions are made.
- People have time for each other.
- Respect is accorded to individuals irrespective of their position in the hierarchy.
- Each member of the team is valued.
- There is absence of threat.

Communicating in writing

A variety of information concerning patients, incidents on the ward, the progress of student nurses and the like has to be communicated in writing. There are a few principles that can be applied, namely:

- Be simple and clear.
- Avoid jargon and meaningless words.
- Be concise and to the point.

- Use technical terminology and language only where appropriate and in the right context.
- Be accurate.
- Do not believe that long words make the piece better.
- Think of the next person who has to understand what has been written.
- In nursing records, convey a portrait of the person, his problems or needs and the nursing given to achieve the goals. The outcomes and evaluation should also be recorded.

Counselling in nursing

Counselling is a familiar and much used term, often adopted in error to describe information giving (see Fig. 4.10).

Fig. 4.10   Giving information to patients (Source: Edwards and Brilhart 1981)

- Use the most specific terms possible with which the patient is likely to be familiar.
- Use words that refer to sensory experience in describing appearance, smell, texture, sound, movement and the feel of bodily sensitivities.
- Reiterate especially important points, rephrasing them in one or more ways with synonyms, i.e. it is like ...'
- Put details in order; what will happen first, second, and so on.
- Encourage the listener to stop you and ask questions regarding anything that is not understood.
- Always respond gladly to any request to clarify: you want the person to understand.
- Compare new ideas and experiences to those with which the person is familiar.

In contrast, counselling refers to a supportive, helping relationship, the task of counselling being to give the client an opportunity to explore, discover, and clarify ways of living more resourcefully and towards greater well-being (Rugby cited in Tschudin 1982). Thus it means that one person can tell his story and another is there to listen and to hear it (Tschudin 1982). The nurse needs to use all her communication skills but in particular listening skills. Effective listening is fundamental so that the nurse hears not only what is said but also what is not mentioned. This process requires self-awareness on the part of the nurse so that she is in a position to facilitate the patient's increasing understanding of himself. The counsellor (i.e. the nurse) needs to show empathy and respect, to be genuine and to use clear language (ibid 1982). In addition, several studies have demonstrated that non-verbal communication skills are important in maximising the effectiveness of these factors in the counselling situation (Rozelle *et al.* 1986).

Counselling contrasts with information giving in that the nurse does not provide the answers.The patient gives himself an answer to his own problems (Tschudin 1982). Nurses may feel tempted to sort out the patient's problem, especially as nursing may be seen as being essentially about 'doing' things. The nurse, however, cannot take on the responsibility for, and solve, all the patient's problems. Indeed, in counselling, even the patient may not find a solution. Working at the problem, however, may be a satisfaction in itself. Tschudin (1982) writes that 'what is happening may constantly elude the patient but if he can see one step ahead of himself then half the battle is won; he will have to take that step himself because no-one else can take it for him'. She goes on to record that the nurse has to:

- listen;
- encourage;
- understand;
- nurture;
- give space;
- allow the patient to 'let go';
- believe what he says.

In interpreting what is not said she also has to use her intuition and be open to what the patient wishes to discuss. This includes difficult subjects such as pain and death. The patient deserves the nurse's individual attention. Thus Rogers (1975) writes of counselling,

> If I can create a relationship characterised on my part by a genuineness and transparency, in which I am my real feelings; by a warm acceptance of and prizing of the other person as a separate individual; by a sensitive ability to see his world and himself as he sees them then the other individual in the relationship:
> - will experience and understand aspects of himself which previously he has repressed
> - will find himself becoming better integrated, more able to function effectively
> - will become more similar to the person he would like to be
> - will be more self-directing and self-confident
> - will become more of a person, more unique and more self-expressive
> - will be more understanding, more acceptant of others
> - will be able to cope with the problems of life more adequately and more comfortably.

Counselling requires tact and patience and has to be learned and practised in order that the skills can be utilised to the benefit of patients, and their families, as well as peers and colleagues. This may be accomplished to a certain degree in the classroom setting using workshops and role play and in the clinical setting by working with and observing other more experienced nurses. Counselling skills may be required in a variety of situations, for example in helping a person who has to come to a decision about treatment or supporting bereaved relatives. However, some situations require high-level counselling skills and the nurse needs to be aware of occasions when referral to a trained counsellor is necessary.

Patient education

There is an increasing amount of research in nursing which provides evidence to suggest that giving patients information concerning their operations and investigations can reduce their subsequent pain and/or stress. Wilson-Barnett (1978) studied the effect of informing patients about their forthcoming barium X-rays on their subsequent emotional reaction to the procedure. A sample of seventy patients who were undergoing barium enemas and fifty-eight having a barium meal was used. A group of patients who received information were compared with a group of patients who did not. Wilson-Barnett (1978) found that although explanation did not effect a significant reduction in the anxiety of patients going for a barium meal it was associated with a reduced anxiety during the barium enema investigation.

Similarly Hayward (1975) sought to test the hypothesis that 'patients who were given information appertaining to their illness and recovery would, when compared to an appropriate control group, report less anxiety and pain during the post-operative recovery period'. He investigated patients in two hospitals. A variety of tools were used including an anxiousness inventory, patient subjective scales of pain and the like, a measure of post-operative analgesic consumption and an assessment of patient's post-operative vomiting. Sisters were then asked to rate the post-operative progress of each patient. Information which had previously been identified as lacking was given to the experimental group. This covered: hospital matters generally; ward practice; pre-operative procedures; pain and discomfort aspects. This type of pre-operative information did indeed reduce the post-operative pain and anxiety (Hayward 1975).

Following on from this Boore (1978) also investigated the relationship between information and recovery. Her patients, eighty in total, were given information similar to that described by Hayward (1975). In addition, patients were taught a selection of post-operative exercises; how to inspire and expire fully, to cough following inspiration and how to reduce pain by supporting the operation wound when coughing. Foot, ankle and leg exercises and the relaxation of abdominal muscles were also included. Several factors were assessed including the patient's physical and mental state and pain. Medical and nursing assessments were made just prior to discharge in order to evaluate the patient's post-operative recovery.

Boore (1978) found that 'the pre-operative giving of information about prospective treatments and care, and the teaching of exercises to be performed post-operatively, will minimise the rise in biochemical indicators of stress'. The implication of this study for the nurse is that informing patients pre-operatively about hospital matters, ward practices, giving the patient a realistic appraisal of pre-operative procedures and the likely post-operative recovery, including details of pain, analgesia and intravenous infusions reduces post-operative pain and stress.

Thinking of patients in the longer term Webb (1983) conducted a study to describe patients' experiences in the first four months following hysterectomy. She tried to assess the influence of personality variables and social support on recovery, as well as to evaluate the effect of an experimental counselling session. During this, information was given to patients and their possible experiences after discharge were discussed. Interestingly, patients who participated in this session did not recall more information than the others. Indeed, Webb (1983) concludes that 'large numbers of women in this study could not remember having been told about their operation beforehand or being prepared for discharge [implying that] what may have been told to them made so little impression that the occasion was not remembered'. When asked what advice they would have liked, most responses concerned activities, what to do or avoid, and warning about the symptoms which had occurred during recovery. As Webb (1983) recommends, 'nurses, whose closeness to patients in terms of contact time and rapport should give them rich opportunities for teaching . . . need to exploit these advantages in a way which really reaches through to patients and helps them to achieve their full recovery potential'.

In considering patient education the nurse has once again to capitalise on all her communication skills. Education demands more than the giving of information. The nurse has to find out what the patient needs and has to assess what the patient has learned from her. Thus the principles of teaching and learning outlined in Chapter 6 can be brought into play. As Wilson-Barnett and Osborne (1984) observe: throughout the patient's stay 'nurses have a responsibility to choose the most helpful aspects to teach, to avoid over-loading or confusing patients and ensuring that it is seen as important to them . . . information which guides the patient through his experience in hospital is necessary'.

The use of touch in nursing

An important aspect of communication is the judicious use of touch. Touch has a variety of meanings for different people according to factors such as cultural background, mood and the nature of the relationship (Tobiason 1981). In Western culture touch is not much used and may be open to misinterpretation. Touching may invade a person's personal space. There may be associated discomfort or embarrassment from the nurse or patient. Despite these problems touch can be used to communicate and may contribute to the plan of the nursing intervention to meet individual needs.

Nurse–patient touch may be classified in two catgegories. 'Instrumental touch' is defined as intentional physical contact while another task is being performed. In contrast 'expressive touch' is spontaneous and affective and is not required as part of another task, e.g. touch used to comfort a distressed patient (Watson 1975 cited by Porter *et al.* 1986) and may include stroking, holding and hugging. McCorkle (1974) demonstrated that touch can be used to enable the nurse to establish a rapport with a seriously ill patient within a short period of time and can communicate that she cares. Indeed, the more traumatic the environment the more important human contact seems to be (Lynch 1978). There are six major tactile symbols to be considered (Weiss 1979), namely:

● duration;
● location;
● action;
● intensity;
● frequency;
● sensation.

Langland and Panicucci (1982) in the United States carried out a small study to examine the effects of touch combined with a verbal request on communication between elderly confused women and a nurse. Thirty-two women were divided into experimental and control groups and their reactions observed. It was found that touching the patients lightly on the forearm while asking them to pick an item increased the patient's attention (non-verbal responses). However, there was not a greater verbal response nor an increase in appropriate action. The conclusion was made that touch here increased the relationship aspect of communication even though no significant increase in reaction to the content aspect was observed.

Despite the importance of touch and the variety of meanings that can be conveyed, evidence suggests (Le May and Redfern 1989) that nurses use much less expressive touch compared with instrumental touch – a deficit that could be remedied as part of the planned care for each individual person. The newly registered nurse might examine her own attitudes to, and use of, touch in order to capitalise on it as a means of communication with patients.

Conclusion

Communication is an interpersonal skill and an integral part of life which can be used to enhance the quality of nursing and yet which can pose difficulties for the nurse. However, in common with other aspects of nursing, a systematic approach to assessing, planning and implementing communication skills to meet patients' individual needs is required. Indeed, as has been illustrated, there are strategies that can be identified and used to the benefit of patients. Nurse–patient interaction is nevertheless only one facet of the nurse's role in relation to communication. It affects every part of her working life, and defines her relationships with others while at the same time being dependent upon them. Some of the issues inherent in this complex process have been raised in this chapter. However, recommendations for good practice to overcome some of the difficulties should not be viewed in isolation from influences that each individual brings to the situation when communicating with another person.

References

Argyle, M. (1969) *Social Interaction*, London: Tavistock Publications.
Ashworth, P. (1980) *Care to Communicate*, London: RCN.
Authier, J., Authier, K. and Lutey, K. (1979) 'Clinical management of the tearfully depressed patient', *Journal of Psychiatric Nursing and Mental Health Services*, Vol. 17 (2), Feb., pp. 34–41.
Beanlands, H. E. and MacKay, R.C. (1981) 'Nurse do you hear me?' *The Canadian Nurse*, Vol. 77 (7), Jul/Aug. pp. 41–3.
Bond, M. (1986) *Stress and Self-awareness: A guide for nurses*, London: William Heinemann Medical Books.
Boore, J. (1978) *Prescription for Recovery*, London: RCN.
Bradley, J. C. and Edinberg, M. A. (1982) *Communication in the Nursing Context*, New York: Appleton Century Crofts.
Bridge, W. and Macleod Clark, J. (1981) 'Nursing and communication', in Bridge, W. and Macleod, Clark, J. (eds.) *Communication in Nursing Care*, London: HM and M Publishers Ltd.
Darbyshire, P. (1987) 'Sour grapes', *Nursing Times*, Vol. 83 (37), pp. 23–5.
DHSS (1984) *Patients Dying in Hospital*, London: DHSS Circular DA (84)17.
Edwards, B. J. and Brilhart, J. (1981) *Communication in Nursing Pratice*, St Louis, Missouri: C.V. Mosby.
Footitt, B. (1981) 'Communicating . . . not just a one-way process', *Nursing Focus*, Vol. 2, (6), pp. 186, 188–9.
French, H. P. (1979) 'Reassurance – a nursing skill?' *Journal of Advanced Nursing*, Vol. 4 (6), pp. 627–34.

Fritz, P. A., Russell, C., Wilcox, E. and Shirk, F. (1984) 'Interpersonal Communication' in *Nursing: An interactionist approach*, Norwalk, Connecticut: Appleton Century Crofts.

Hacking, M. (1981) 'Communicating with dying patients and their relatives', In Bridge, W. and Macleod Clark, J. (eds.) *Communication in Nursing Care*, London: HM & M Publishers, Ch. 9, pp. 133–55.

Hargie, O. and Marshall, P. (1986) 'Interpersonal communication: A theoretical framework', in Hargie, O. (ed.) *A Handbook of Communication Skills*, Beckenham, Kent: Croom Helm.

Hayward, J. (1975) *Information – a Prescription Against Pain*, London: RCN.

Heineken, J. and Roberts, F. (1983) 'Confirming, not disconfirming: Communicating in a more positive manner' *MCN American Journal of Maternal/Child Nursing*, Vol. 8(1), Jan./Feb., pp. 78–80.

Hinton, J. (1974) *Dying,* Harmondsworth: Penguin.

Kelly, M. P. and May, D. (1982) 'Good and bad patients: a review of the literature and a theoretical critique'. *Journal of Advanced Nursing,* Vol. 7 (2), pp. 147–56.

Knight, M. and Field, D. (1981) 'A silent conspiracy: coping with dying patients on an acute surgical ward', *Journal of Advanced Nursing*, Vol. 6, pp. 221–9.

Langland, R. M. and Panicucci, C. L. (1982) 'Effects of touch on communication with elderly confused clients', *Journal of Gerontological Nursing*, Vol. 8 (3), pp. 152–5.

Lay, T. N. (1979) 'Personal awareness: Therapeutic communication', *The Journal of Nursing Care*, Vol. 12 (9), Sep., pp. 16–18.

Le May, A. and Redfern, S. (1989) 'Touch and elderly people', in Wilson-Barnett, J. and Robinson, S. (eds.) *Directions in Nursing Research*, London: Scutari Press.

Lynch, J. L. (1978) 'The simple act of touching', *Nursing (USA)*, Vol. 8 (6), pp. 32–6.

Macleod Clark, J. (1984) 'Verbal communication in nursing', in Faulkner, A. (ed.) *Recent Advances in Nursing: Communication (7)*, Edinburgh: Churchill Livingstone, Ch. 3, pp. 53–73.

Maguire, P. (1985) 'Consequences of poor communication between nurses and patients', *Nursing*, Vol. 2 (36), pp. 1115–18.

Marshall, P. D. (1985) 'Nursing patients – an enjoyable task?' *Journal of Advanced Nursing*, Vol. 10 (5), pp. 429–34.

McCorkle, R. (1974) 'Effects of touch on seriously ill patients', *Nursing Research*, Vol. 23 (2), 125–32.

McMorrow, M. E. (1981) 'The manipulative patient', *American Journal of Nursing*, Vol. 81 (6), pp. 1188–90.

Melia, K. (1987) 'Everyday ethics for nurses: justice for all'. *Nursing Times*, Vol. 83 (31) pp. 43–5.

Porter, L., Redfern, S., Wilson-Barnett, J. and Le May, A. (1986) 'The development of an observation schedule for measuring nurse–patient touch, using an ergonomic approach', *International Journal of Nursing Studies*, Vol. 23 (1), pp. 11–20.

Roberts, D. (1984) 'Non-verbal communication', in Faulkner, A. (ed.). *Recent Advances in Nursing Communication*, Edinburgh: Churchill Livingstone, Ch.1, pp. 3–28.

Rogers, C. (1975) *On Becoming a Person*, London: Constable.

Roper, N., Logan, W. and Tierney, A. (1980) *The Elements of Nursing*, Edinburgh: Churchill Livingstone.

Rozelle, R., Druckman, D. and Baxter, J. (1986) 'Non-verbal communication', in Hargie, O. (ed.) *A Handbook of Communication Skills*, Beckenham, Kent: Croom Helm, Ch. 3, pp. 59–94.

Runciman, P. (1983) *Ward Sister at Work*, Edinburgh: Churchill Livingstone.

Shields, P. (1984) 'Communication: A supportive bridge between cancer patient, family and health care staff'. *Nursing Forum*, Vol. 21 (1), pp. 31–6.

Shuldham, C. M. (1984) 'Communication – a conscious effort', *Nursing*, Vol. 2 (23) pp. 673–5.

Stockwell, F. (1972) *The Unpopular Patient*, London: RCN.

Tobiason, S. J. B. (1981) 'Touching is for everyone', *American Journal of Nursing*, Vol. 81 (4), pp. 728–30.

Trockman, G. (1978) 'Caring for the confused or delirious patient', *American Journal of Nursing*, Vol. 78 (9), pp. 1495–9.

Tschudin, V. (1982) *Counselling Skills for Nurses*, London; Bailliere Tindall.

Walton, I. (1986) 'Lessons from the health service; Ombudsman's report'. *Nursing Times Occasional Paper*, Vol. 82 (10) 2, July pp. 54–7.

Webb, C. (1983) 'A study of recovery from hysterectomy,' in Wilson-Barnett, J. (ed.) *Nursing Research: Ten Studies in Patient Care*, Chichester: John Wiley & Sons, Ch. 10, pp. 195-228.

Weiss, S, (1979) 'The language of touch', *Nursing Research,* Vol. 28 (2) pp. 76–80.

West, T. S., Kirkham, S. R. (1983) 'The family', in Saunders, C., Summers, D. and Teller, N. (eds.) *Hospice: 'the living idea'*, London: Edward Arnold, Ch. 2 'Hospice as a style for living: the family', pp. 19–66, 47.

Wilson-Barnett, J. (1978) 'Patients' emotional responses to barium X-rays'. *Journal of Advanced Nursing*, Vol 3(1), pp. 37–46.

Wilson-Barnett, J. and Osborne, J. (1983) 'Studies evaluating patient teaching', *International Journal of Nursing Studies*, Vol. 20 (1), pp. 33–44,

5 Teaching and Learning

ANGELA HESLOP AND JUDITH LATHLEAN

Introduction

While teaching is an important part of the registered nurse's role, many feel inhibited and ill-prepared for the task; some do not see themselves as teachers but, rather, as managers or clinicians. This is often due to a narrow view of what teaching is, a limited understanding of how people learn, and a lack of well-developed skills. Thus it is useful, first, to consider the principles and theories which underlie the processes by which people learn to nurse and how they develop expertise within nursing and, second, the different factors that contribute to effective teaching and learning in the clinical area and in the creation of a climate that is conducive for learning.

Project 2000 is having a great impact on the teaching role of the staff nurse in focusing on them as mentors to supernumerary students. This key role – welcomed by some and daunting to others – is explored, including some of the strategies that can be useful such as learning contracts and learning by reflecting on action. Alongside this, the evaluation of learning has become an even more important topic; thus approaches to assessment are discussed. However, not all nurses will be mentoring students, especially when the nurse is newly registered. Although they may feel that teaching is not part of their role, there are many ways in which they can facilitate learning for others as well as increase their own knowledge and understanding. A number of learning opportunities are considered in this chapter, whereas Chapter 9 looks specifically at the professional development needs of the newly registered nurse herself.

Approaches to learning

The definition of learning has been a source of controversy – there is no single theory to account for all aspects of learning. Whilst some theorists have described learning as a relatively permanent *change* in behaviour (for example, Hilgard and Atkinson 1967), others have suggested that the term can be use to encompass 'the acquisition of new knowledge, skill or attitude by study, experience or teaching' (Jarvis 1983). There is general agreement that there are three main approaches to learning: behavioural; humanistic; and cognitive. Some (for example, Quinn 1988) also include social learning theory as an important approach. In addition, Moore (1989) adds a fifth to this list, that of the theory of andragogy (the art and science of helping adults learn) whereas others (for example, Jarvis and Gibson 1985) consider adult learning as a subject in its own right rather than as an approach to, or theory of learning.

Behavioural approaches

The terms 'behavioural' or 'behaviourist' are used to cover a range of different approaches, the essence of which is the explanation of learning in terms of stimulus and response with an emphasis on a *change* of behaviour. The work of Pavlov (1960), a physiologist, illustrated the principles of 'classic conditioning' by showing that a dog could be made to salivate at the sound of a bell, as long as the sound had on several previous occasions been presented simultaneously with food. This kind of instant reflex action can be apparent in emergency situations, when it seems to the individual that she is reacting 'instinctively' to a response such as a cardiac arrest, or an alarm bell on a cardiac monitor. However, it may be the result of classic conditioning – an automatic response to a certain stimulus.

Thorndike's (1928) research showed that learning occurs through trial and error, and that behaviour which results in success or reward is more likely to occur than behaviour which does not. Thorndike concluded that repetition of meaningful actions led to substantial learning. The implications of this for nursing are that the greater the pleasure obtained from the learning experience, the more learning that will occur, and that 'practice makes perfect'. However, possibly the most pervasive influence on behaviourist theories has been the work of the psychologist Skinner (1953). He developed a theory of operant conditioning by demonstrating that rats and pigeons could be taught desirable behaviours by rewarding the correct behaviour at each step in the development. This is different from Pavlov's notions of stimulus and response because with operant conditioning reinforcement (i.e. reward) is used to modify the behaviour.

Some people argue that behavioural theory may not be appropriate for human learning because most of the original research was undertaken with animals. However, over the years, it has been widely used to describe how people learn. The idea of operant conditioning has been influential in 'programmed learning' which was popular in nurse education in the 1950s and 1960s, and behavioural theory in general has had a significant impact on nurse training, particularly in relation to the use of behavioural objectives and the development of nursing skills (for further discussion see Moore 1989).

Cognitive approaches

A second general approach is that of the cognitive theorists. Within this, the Gestalt psychologists argued that people perceive things as wholes rather than as parts of the whole and that individuals grasp patterns of action when seeking to solve a problem. From this it has been concluded that solutions to problems seem to come about by inspiration or insight (the so-called 'aha' syndrome), and that they occur as a result of the individual perceiving certain relationships. The implication for learning is that it is beneficial for a person to be offered a meaningful whole first, rather than a series of seemingly disparate parts. So if a nurse is teaching some aspect of nursing she should show the 'learner' what she is aiming for, before proceeding to explain the parts.

Others using cognitive approaches include Ausubel (1978) who argues that learning occurs by the interaction of new information with the cognitive processes that an individual already has, and suggests that the teacher use an advance organiser – that is, general ideas which provide an overview and prelude to later more detailed material. There are many examples in nurse education where, first, the teacher presents the most general ideas and then moves on to the detail and, second, the teacher tries to find out the level of the student's previous knowledge and understanding in order to judge how to move on to new information, and then consciously relates all new ideas to previously learnt ones.

Social learning theory

Social learning theorists, for example Bandura (1977), suggest that individuals learn *all* behaviour by observing others, the idea of role modelling. Certainly, research has shown that *one* way in which nurses learn how to behave is through a process of identification with role models. For example, Pembrey (1980) in her study of ward sisters found that the 'manager' sisters named other senior sisters as a source of their learning and Marson (1981) found that student nurses were influenced by staff nurses and sisters who possessed qualities that were valued by the students, such as having high standards and showing care and concern for the patients.

Humanist approaches

Humanistic theories have been developed in direct contrast to the behaviourist theories and the psychologists supporting this approach, such as Maslow and Rogers, have stressed the control that an individual has over his environment and his learning. The theories suggest that what a person does and how he learns is very influenced by his inner states and his aspirations. Maslow (1970) and Rogers (1983) place emphasis on the learner being at the centre of their own learning process. The key features of this approach, as identified by Rogers (1969), can be summarised as follows:

1. Individuals have a natural drive to learn, particularly if the learning is seen as enhancing an individual's self-concept;
2. Learning is best achieved in certain conditions such as:
   - a trusting and non-threatening climate,
   - through experience,
   - when the teacher and student mutually participate at all stages,
   - when feelings and intellect are involved,
   - when self-evaluation is encouraged (after Moore 1989).

There has been much research undertaken which supports these beliefs. For example, Fretwell (1982) found that for learning to take place on the ward, the environment needed to be thought of as non-threatening and there needed to be mutual participation in learning. Indeed, the ideas of the humanists have been very pervasive in nurse education in recent years and have been important in such developments as student centred approaches to learning (see, for example, McEvoy 1989).

While all these theories can be seen to have relevance for teaching and learning in nursing, behavioural approaches have perhaps been the most influential in the past, and humanist approaches more recently. Table 5.1 compares these two approaches.

Nevertheless, nursing is a complex mixture of learning activities, encompassing knowledge, skills and attitudes acquired and experienced in a variety of settings. To achieve learning in the formal sense, planned teaching needs to be based on well-designed curricula which often have explicit or implicit behavioural objectives. In addition, the nurse will learn from various different teachers who are particularly knowledgeable about or experienced in certain areas, from good role models, and through her own self-directed means. This should be coupled with appropriate and relevant assessment and regular feedback about progress made. So it can be seen that a combination of these approaches is relevant in the ward setting.

Adult learning

Much attention has been paid in recent years to the differences between the way in which adults and children learn. Knowles (1970), an educator, has developed a, now well-known, theory of andragogy – adult learning – which is based on the following four assumptions:

1. *The learner's self concept:* the learner moves from dependence to

Table 5.1 Comparison of two approaches to learning

Theory	Type of learning			Method
Behavioural	Teacher centred	Achievement of objectives	Teacher as expert	
	Teacher decides what should be learnt and teaches it	Learning is judged by the achievement of set objectives – the outcome is all important	Teacher imparts knowledge – teacher knows more than student	Emphasis on formal lectures and formal instruction – didactic teaching
Humanist	Student centred	Learning by discovery	Teacher as facilitator	
	Student identifies for herself what she wants to know and actively pursues this	The process of learning is as important as the outcome	Teacher shares knowledge with the student and facilitates learning	Mix of methods: lectures, seminars, experiential (such as role play, projects, etc.) with feedback to and from the teacher

independence during maturation. The implications of this are that adults have a need to be self-directing in their learning and thus the role of the teacher is to engage in a process of mutual enquiry with them rather than to transmit his or her knowledge to them and then evaluate their conformity to it. Emphasis is placed on the person diagnosing her own learning needs which is done in collaboration with the teacher, and in planning with the teacher how these needs can be met. Self-assessment is encouraged and the learner achieves this by collecting evidence about her progress.

2. *The learner's experiences:* the actual experiences of the learner can in themselves become an increasingly rich source for learning. This means that methods which make use of the experience, such as experiential learning, tend to be preferred. (For an overview of experiential learning see Miles 1987.) Also, there should be opportunities for putting the learning into practice.

3. *The learner's readiness to learn:* adults are ready to learn material which will enable them to perform more effectively in some aspects of their lives (Knowles 1984). Therefore it is more appropriate to study life or work situations rather than discrete subjects.

4. *The learner's orientation to learning:* adults enter learning with an interest in solving problems and gaining knowledge which will be of use to them in their

working and personal lives. This implies that learning should have the learner at the centre, that the expectations of the learner should be explored, and that the learning experience should be concerned with solving problems.

Knowles has been criticised on the grounds that his work is not based on research. Nevertheless, many of the principles do appear to have some validity in practice, and there is a good deal of evidence to suggest they are influencing nurse education as shown by the increasing use of, for example, learning contracts and self-assessment techniques. These will be discussed later in the chapter.

Learning from experience in nursing

A number of researchers have turned their attention in recent years to the idea that experience is an important part of learning the job of nursing. Indeed, everyday experience in clinical nursing practice is considered to be essential to developing knowledge and skills – or expertise – as nursing is a practice-based profession (UKCC 1987). Several studies have examined the learning which occurs in experience in clinical practice. For example, Lathlean *et al.* (1986) distinguished between two types of experience, experience *per se*, which happened merely as a result of working as a registered nurse, and experience with specific conditions or features which facilitated learning, such as working alongside a more experienced nurse. Lathlean *et al.* concluded that the second type of experience was more likely to result in learning than the first.

This research finding is supported by the work of Farnish (1983) who studied how well sisters felt prepared for their roles and what they considered to be their major sources of learning as staff nurses. Learning by experience was cited, but Farnish identified this as a 'hit and miss' approach – they may or may not learn aspects that were of use to them in their subsequent roles as sisters. Furthermore, both experience and role modelling have their limitations as they are likely to reinforce the status quo, irrespective of the quality of care provided.

Experiential learning, which is increasingly being used in nurse education (see, for example, Major 1989), focuses on the links between learning and experience. There are a number of different approaches which come under the general title of experiental learning. One of the foremost is that devised by Kolb and Fry (1975) which can be depicted as shown in Fig. 5.1. According to Kolb (1984), experience is vital for learning, but just having the experience *alone* is not enough for learning to occur – it needs to be observed and reflected upon. As the person reflects upon or thinks about the experience he develops 'theories' which can be used in new situations. So if, for example, a nurse reflects on how she handled a difficult situation with a grieving relative, she

Fig. 5.1 Experiential learning

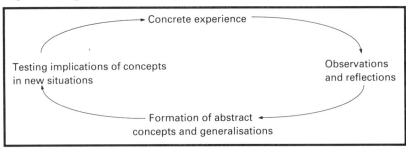

might 'abstract' from this that listening and showing her own emotions appeared to be helpful, and that such behaviour might be useful in the future in similar situations. The suggestion is that the nurse only learns from that experience if she consciously stands back, and examines her thoughts, feelings, actions and conclusions. Boud *et al.* (1985) also say that learning from experience only really takes place if the experience is recalled, described and 'processed'.

The idea of the *reflective practitioner* has been developed both in teacher education (George 1987) and in the education of a number of different professionals including architects, teachers, psychiatrists and managers (Argyris and Schön 1974, and Schön 1983). It also seems to be relevant to nursing. Schön (1983) argues that competent, experienced professionals are reflective practitioners in that they engage in 'reflection-in-action'. This process involves becoming conscious of their own tacit 'knowledge', the knowledge that informs their actions but which is normally just taken for granted. This 'knowledge' is then subjected to critical examination as it is used to make new sense of situations of uncertainty and uniqueness. Schön suggests that the practitioner has a 'reflective conversation with the situation', teasing out the norms and ideas underlying action and the way the problem is defined or 'framed'. He or she then reframes the problem, draws on a repertoire of similar problems and analogous experiences, develops new hypotheses and tests them out, either in the mind or in reality. It is suggested that there are different ways in which this process of reflection can be useful for many professions; for example, the experienced professional can make available to the clients and to others the new insights gained from the process, and students and novice practitioners can improve their practice by becoming more reflective and thus learning from their practice.

Powell (1989), in a small-scale study of eight practising registered nurses, explored their use of reflection-in-action in their everyday work. She concluded that 'reflection-in-action [was] present extensively in the form of description and of planning of actions, but to a lesser extent in the area of recognition of value judgments and the areas of reflection-in-action leading to learning taking place. Where these were found, albeit in small quantities, they were almost exclusively confined to the community nurses and the nurse practitioner.' These nurses were also much more aware than the others of the potential of learning from everyday practice.

It appears, then, that learning from practice can take place where the nurse reflects on that practice. But what is the relationship between that and the development of expertise in nursing? In other words, how do nurses become *expert* nurses? The research of Benner (1984) is valuable here. Benner's notion of how nurses move through stages of performance from novice to expert has already been described in Chapter 2. The research shows that expertise (i.e. practical knowledge) is gained by repeated encounters with particular situations or in caring for particular kinds of patients over a very long period of time; from these the nurse builds up her 'know how'. But the expert nurses found it difficult to articulate *how* they knew, and why they were skilled practitioners, saying such things as 'it felt right' or 'it looked good'. The findings imply that if ways can be found of gaining access to this embedded knowledge, possibly by a process of reflection and analysis, then this could be passed on to other, less experienced nurses, which could be very beneficial.

MacLeod (1990) also set out to explore the topic of expertise. She studied ten surgical ward sisters who had been identified as excellent, experienced clinical nurses and found that their everyday experience appeared much more complex and fluid than the empirical literature suggests. The 'sisters' moment-by-moment practices . . . emerged as purposeful, complex, multi-faceted and patient-centred. Underlying these practices, a process of noticing, understanding and acting could be discerned.' She found the sisters to be attuned to experience – their own, other people's and, crucially, the patients. She concluded that being attuned to experience is critical to developing expertise in practice and that expertise is relational and context-specific.

In conclusion, at the heart of much of this thinking is the interest in the relationship between the 'theory' and the 'practice' of nursing, and the concern, particularly in nurse education, about the gap between theoretical knowledge and practical experience. Many people are attempting both to understand the two and to try to draw them closer together. Lathlean and Vaughan (forthcoming) review the underlying issues and describe some ways in which people have tried to overcome the problems.

Facilitating learning in clinical settings

The discussion so far has centred on the theory of how people – particularly adults – learn, and it has been suggested that different approaches may well be appropriate for different purposes and in various situations. The way in which people learn from practice has also been explored. Since the staff nurse will mainly be involved in teaching on the ward or in other clinical settings it is useful to review some of the factors that appear to inhibit or promote learning from practice. Two main aspects will be considered: the importance of the learning environment; and different approaches to teaching.

The learning environment

It is now well acknowledged that clinical areas have a 'climate' or atmosphere that can help or hinder learning. This facet seems to be important to many nurses. For example, Jacka and Lewin (1987) asked students to list those aspects that assisted their learning most and the most frequently cited item was ward atmosphere. Orton (1981) found that ward learning climate exists as a reality for student nurses and that it can be measured. Orton refers in her research to high and low student orientation wards; the hallmark of high student orientation wards was the combination of teamwork, consultation and the sister's awareness of the physical and emotional needs of her staff. In addition, emphasis was laid on learners as learners and not merely as pairs of hands. Individualised care for patients tended to be the norm. Fretwell (1980) also undertook research which showed that a good learning environment existed where the ward was not hierarchical, where teamwork, negotiation and good communication were prevalent and where trained staff were 'facilitators' of learning rather than teachers. Reid (1986) showed that a ward which takes an individualised approach to the care of patients offers a better learning environment for the student nurse.

The role of the sister in creating a climate that is conducive for learning has been stressed. For example, in studying the leadership style of sisters, Ogier (1982) developed a 'tool' for completion by students, called the 'Learner's Perception of Ward Climate', one of the purposes of which was to distinguish between ward sisters who were 'ideal' for nurse learners and those who were not. Two of the key indicators were found to be sisters who were interested in the students and sisters who helped them.

Conversely, what factors in a ward climate inhibit learning? The nurse who feels a passive member of the team, who does not consider that her education and experience are relevant and who is discouraged from thinking is less likely to learn. As she copes with sick and distressed people she learns more about herself, but this in turn may lead to anxiety about coping with the situation. Too much or too little responsibility for the newly registered nurse can militate against learning as can a heavy workload (Jacka and Lewin 1987).

Approaches to teaching

There appear to be as many definitions of teaching as there are of learning, and most of these refer to a formal teaching role where the teacher teaches and the learner learns. Indeed, many definitions include the words 'tell', 'instruct' or 'inform'. Ogier (1982) explored the meaning of the term 'teaching' with groups of students and trained staff, and the majority described didactic situations where teachers imparted knowledge and learners sat in front of them, or where the teacher was demonstrating a skill. Yet in a clinical setting learning occurs in a number of different ways, and through a variety of different means, the formal 'imparting of knowledge' being only a part. Rogers (1969) suggests that it is preferable to use the term 'facilitator' rather than 'teacher', and it is certainly through the process of facilitation that much clinical learning occurs. So, for example, when acting as a facilitator the nurse may well not be telling the learner how to do some aspect of nursing, or even showing her, with the emphasis being on the nurse's greater knowledge and expertise. Rather, she may be providing the opportunity for someone else to observe her, and talk with her, with both sharing their knowledge and ideas.

There has been some work on what makes a good teacher, using the term 'teacher' in the sense of facilitator. Based on her research, Marson (1981) suggests that the qualities of good 'teachers' fall into four broad areas: the role model; managerial styles; interpersonal behaviours; and instructional skills. The theorists have suggested that modelling one's behaviour upon others is an important way of learning and it does seem that in this respect behaviour may speak louder than words. One of the aspects of being a mentor is that of role modelling and therefore it is important for nurses to be aware of the effect they have on other people – students and trained staff. Exercise 5.1 can be used to identify the important aspects.

Interpersonal skills such as empathy and sensitivity to the needs of learners are necessary qualities of good 'teachers' (Marson 1981), as are consideration and warmth (Ogier 1982). Good teachers are also considered to be good managers in being seen to organise their work and, in the case of ward sisters, the ward well. Formal teaching skills were also mentioned in Marson's study but not with the same frequency as the other three categories.

Rogers (1969) suggests that a good teacher will:

- communicate trust in the students;
- help students to clarify their personal and group objectives;
- assume that students are motivated;
- act as a resource person in showing what learning experiences are available;
- be a resource person to individuals;
- learn to recognise emotional messages among the students;
- be open in expressing his/her feelings with the group;
- have empathy in relation to the group's feelings;
- finally, know him/herself.

Exercise 5.1   Learning from role models

Learning from other people

Think of a recent example where you were impressed by the way in which someone else undertook a particular task or activity. (This could be a clinical procedure; the way someone dealt with a situation; an aspect of communication, etc.)

- What was it about the incident/event that you thought was positive?
- What was it about the person, for example, their behaviour, their skill, their personality, their position that contributed to the positive action?
- What have you learnt from observing this incident/event?

Then repeat the same type of questions – but for a task or activity that you thought was poorly handled. Substitute negative for positive in the second and third questions.

Other people learning from me

Think of a recent example where you were aware that other people/ another person was observing what you were doing.

- How do you feel about the fact that other people are observing you, e.g. anxious; aware but see it as a positive thing; very confident?

What strengths do you have that you feel others can learn from?
What weaknesses do you have that you feel other people should avoid copying?
What ways can you think of to help others learn from you?

These qualities seem to dovetail with the kinds of characteristics that the aforementioned research has identified.

The role of the nurse as mentor

With the changes in nurse education, the role of the staff nurse as 'mentor' has come to the fore. The term is not a new one, having derived from Greek mythology. It has achieved more prominence with the implementation of Project 2000, though it was referred to by the English National Board prior to this in its course approval document (ENB 1987). Whilst much has been written about mentors and mentoring, there is no consensus about the definition and there is confusion in these terms between the person, the process, the purposes and the activities and an overlap between this and other roles such as 'supervisor', 'assessor', 'role model' and 'preceptor' (Bradshaw 1989; Donovan 1990). But as Morle (1990) points out, the absence of a clear definition of the role, function and preparation of the mentor does not seem to have hindered the ready uptake of the idea.

What is mentoring?

The Concise Oxford Dictionary defines the word 'mentor' as 'an experienced and trusted advisor', and certainly these two elements feature in some of the other descriptions; for example May (1982) talks about the mentor as someone who is 'knowledgeable and wise in the area'. Others stress the supportive function of mentors; for example, Darling (1984), in posing the question 'what do nurses want in a mentor?' makes the distinction between three different roles: Inspirer ('she sparked my interest in . . .'); Investor ('she saw my capabilities and pushed me'); and Supporter ('she was extremely encouraging'). But a mentor can also have other functions such as assisting in career development (Bracken and Davis 1989) and in easing the transition from a student to staff nurse (Talarczyk and Milbrandt 1988) or other difficult transitions (Daloz 1986). In this respect it is interesting to note that the PREPP document recommends that support should be provided to all newly registered nurses by an experienced nurse, who will be known as a 'preceptor' (rather than a mentor). These people will 'act as role models for newly registered practitioners in day to day practice and with them evolve individual teaching and learning methods' (UKCC 1990).

Daloz (1986) suggests that mentors have three fairly distinct functions: they support; they challenge; and they provide vision. Support refers to 'those acts through which the mentor affirms the validity of the student's present experience' and whereas the function of support is to 'bring boundaries together, challenge peels them apart'. Challenge serves to open a gap between student and environment, a gap that creates tension and calls for closure, and vision offers an idea of what the learner is aiming for. There is a relationship between these three components, as shown in Fig. 5.2.

When support and challenge in mentoring are low, little is likely to happen – things stay much as they are. When support is increased, the learner feels confirmed, that is, good about herself, but it is only when challenge is high as well that growth occurs. Conversely, if there is a good deal of challenge but no support, this can lead to the learner retreating. Finally, if there is high support and challenge plus vision, then real development can take place.

According to Daloz (1986) the suggested elements of these three functions of a mentor are as follows:

Support
- listening;
- giving structure (in that some 'mentees' need specific guidance);

Fig. 5.2   The relationship between different aspects of mentoring
(Adapted from Daloz 1986)

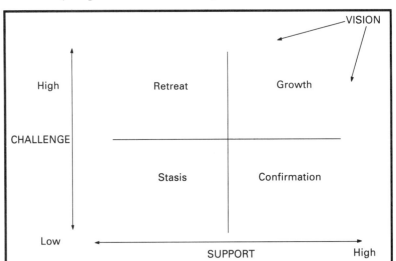

- being positive about expectations;
- being an advocate;
- sharing oneself with the 'mentee';
- making the relationship 'special'.

Challenge
- setting tasks;
- engaging in discussion or 'developmental dialogue';
- creating a pressure for the resolution of dichotomies;
- constructing hypotheses;
- setting high standards.

Vision
- modelling;
- passing on tradition;
- offering a map;
- suggesting new language to describe reality;
- providing a mirror (to reflect the experience of the learner).

This appears to be a useful way of thinking about the multiple roles of mentors.

Perceptions of mentoring

Although there has been quite a good deal written about mentors and descriptions of mentor schemes (for example, Morris *et al.* 1988; Lee 1989) there has as yet been little British research on mentors. However, a small-scale, unpublished study by Atkins (1990) has shown that nurses' perceptions of the role match the wide ranging definitions found in the literature: that a mentor is 'somebody you can go to for professional support', 'a friend', 'someone who teaches clinical skills and assesses', or a 'role model'. The qualities identified for a good mentor have a great deal in common with the qualities of a good teacher, as previously mentioned in the chapter. Thus the mentor should be:

- aware of student needs;
- patient;
- knowledgeable;
- good at setting standards;
- approachable.

Atkins (1990) also asked nurses who were likely to become mentors to students about the satisfactions and dissatisfactions that they felt they might experience. The 'positives' were thought to be:

- working out a strategy together for how to cope with problems;
- seeing progress in the 'mentee';
- sharing knowledge;
- the student's enthusiasm;
- the opportunity to learn from the student.

The potential difficulties were identified as:

- the pressure of time;
- the lack of opportunity to discuss things and reflect with the student;
- the stress of being a mentor and the need to have a break from the role;
- the concern that the student might have needs that could not be met by the mentor;
- the anxiety about being watched closely by someone else.

Mentors in clinical settings

For most registered nurses, the mentor will most likely be seen as the person who relates closely to student nurses and plays a part in their clinical education. The English National Board makes it clear in its documents (for example, ENB 1987 and 1988) that mentorship is a clinical role and one that rests with a qualified first-level nurse. However, it is likely that different institutions will construe that role in different ways according to their particular requirements. Each ward or unit will need to identify criteria for the selection of mentors. For example, it might be specified that only nurses with at least six months' experience will be eligible and/or that nurses will not be expected to act as mentors continuously, the job being rotated among a group of registered nurses on a ward for different 'sets' of students.

The responsibilities and standards expected of mentors should be carefully considered in the light of the needs of students, whether they are supernumerary, the availability, skills, inclinations and needs of the registered nurses and the particular requirements of the programme of nurse education. Whilst it is neither possible nor desirable to have a standard set of activities for all nurses occupying mentor or similar roles, it can be useful to consider the kind of specification that is successfully being used in a health authority. Fig. 5.3 gives one possible role outline, showing the activities and standards expected. It is based on a modified version of an actual specification, that of Oxford Polytechnic in conjunction with Oxfordshire Health Authority.

Preparation for mentors

For mentoring to be effective, mentors need preparation both for the skills of mentoring and for the aspects of the particular programme that they will be involved in. Burnard (1988) suggests that there are certain aspects of the job that are amenable to training, notably skills in identifying learning objectives with the students, interpersonal skills, coaching skills and skills in enabling the student to self-evaluate.

Although the ENB 998 Course on *Teaching and Assessing in Clinical Practice* may seem to be appropriate in developing the mentors' teaching role (Morle 1990), many mentors will have a wider remit than this, and therefore the optimum preparation and support for mentors may need a range of aspects such as on-site meetings of mentors, support groups, and the use of distance learning materials (Wright 1989).

Learning contracts

Whilst learning contracts are not a new phenomena they have been emphasised by the moves within nursing towards more student-centred learning, with the opportunities for students to identify their own needs in relation to the overall objectives and to the competencies that they need to achieve (Jarvis 1986). They can be equally appropriate for students in initial nurse education as for qualified nurses seeking to plan their professional development.

Knowles (1984) identifies the following eight stages in the learning contract from the learner's point of view:

1. Diagnose your learning need.
2. Specify your learning objectives.

Fig. 5.3 The mentor's task: main activities and standards (Adapted from Oxford Polytechnic/Oxfordshire HA Mentor Training Package 1990)

Activities
1. Discuss and agree a contract with the student which identifies the objectives and competencies that the student wants/needs to achieve.
2. Discuss and agree with the student the resources and strategies required for her learning.
3. Plan the learning experiences with the student so that the competencies can be achieved.
4. Encourage self-assessment by the student; personally assess the learning outcomes, ensuring that there is sufficient evidence to support both the student's and the mentor's assessment.
5. Identify and ensure that opportunities are made for the student to reflect on her experiences.
6. Encourage the student to record her experiences as soon as possible after the event in her personal log/diary.
7. Monitor performance as a mentor, e.g. keep written records of time spent with student, and learning opportunities provided for student; record difficulties experienced with the role; discuss the role with the relevant people (e.g. lecturer/practitioner, sister, tutor).

Standards
1. Demonstrate a high standard of professional practice.
2. Demonstrate a breadth of knowledge about the field of practice.
3. Demonstrate personal development of reflective practice.
4. Demonstrate evidence of ongoing awareness of current professional issues and personal development
   - read professional journals at least monthly;
   - negotiate to attend appropriate meetings/study opportunities;
   - reflect on practice and produce action plans.
5. Contribute to developing practice in the area
   - participate in debates about actual practice, health care and health promotion;
   - participate in the systematic evaluation of professional action and in the formulation of plans to improve this.
6. Contribute to enhancing an environment conducive to learning
   - demonstrate foundation level knowledge about the learning process;
   - demonstrate the ability to facilitate learning with the student.

---

3. Specify your learning resources and strategies.
4. Specify what evidence of accomplishment you will be aiming to supply.
5. Specify how the evidence will be validated.

6. Review your contract.
7. Carry out the contract.
8. Evaluate the learning.

The actual format of the learning contract should be based on the needs of the students and the particular situation. One possibility is a fairly open-ended structure which simply specifies the main headings to be considered, such as the objectives and the competencies, the resources and the strategies, and the evidence and standard of achievement. Alternatively, the learning contract can contain much more detail, and include, for example, rating scales. The ENB *Managing Change in Nursing Education* package (ENB 1987) gives guidance on learning contracts and includes useful examples, and Norton (1989) discusses and evaluates the use of contract learning in nurse education.

Assessment

Assessment – both formal and informal – is an important part of the learning process. The registered nurse has a major responsibility for the assessment of students – an activity that is very daunting for some. Nevertheless, this responsibility is being emphasised even more with the implementation of Project 2000 schemes and mentorship schemes.

Assessment strategies

Many new schemes for assessment are being or have been developed in line with changes in nurse education, and whilst each is individual and related to the particular needs of the situation they tend to incorporate some common principles including the following:

- The assessment is based on the achievement of competencies over a wide range of knowledge, skills, attitudes and experiences (e.g. social abilities, communication skills, practical skills and decision-making abilities (Skelton 1989)).
- Different 'levels' of performance are expected in relation to these competencies over time.
- Different types of strategies are used to provide evidence of performance and achievement, for example learning contracts, reflective diaries and methods of student self-assessment. For example, Sigsworth and Heslop (1988) describe the successful use of a 'kard' system for students to record good and bad experiences and events, progress and plans, which can then be used as a basis for discussion.
- The students should play a part in the process, for example by assessing their own performance or by giving themselves a grade which is then discussed with others.

- The process of assessment is continuous rather than based on a final judgement.

Also, although in the past the ward sister has probably been the person with the most involvement with assessment of clinical practice, in the future, the staff nurse – often acting as mentor to the student – will have an important part to play. The following example shows how this might work in a situation where there is either a Project 2000 programme or one where students are supernumerary for all or for most of the time, and where the staff nurse is acting as mentor:

- The student comes to the ward with a list of competencies that she needs to achieve in the course.
- The student discusses the competencies with the mentor, identifies those that she hopes to/needs to achieve during the placement and draws up a learning contract with her, which matches the kind of experience that it is possible to gain during the placement.
- The mentor agrees to work with the student for a minimum number of shifts, and ensures that the necessary resources are available as far as possible.
- The student keeps a reflective diary to record her experiences and fills in the learning contract.
- At the end of the placement, the student discusses her experience with the mentor and usually the ward sister or lecturer practitioner, including the evidence for the achievement of the competencies.
- The mentor and/or sister 'validate' the achievement of the competencies by considering their own observations, alongside the evidence provided by the student.
- The mentor/sister/lecturer practitioner and the student agree one (or more) grades or marks, or the level reached, according to the required system and a pre-set grading profile.

This is only one possibility; the actual process will obviously need to be related to the requirements of the programme. However, it can be seen that such an approach emphasises the responsibility of students for their own learning and the facilitative role of the staff nurse (rather than the judgement role) much more than some traditional systems do. For other examples of assessment approaches, based on the same principles, see Skelton (1989) and Darbyshire et al. (1990).

Opportunities for learning on the ward

As mentioned before, there are many different ways in which nurses can learn in clinical settings; and sometimes various learning opportunities tend to get overlooked. These can be potentially useful for both registered nurses and students. The following are not intended as an exhaustive list but should serve to indicate the diversity of learning situations for both – indeed for anyone who needs to know about the detailed care of patients in that clinical setting.

Handover/reports on patients' conditions

The handover, which usually occurs at shift change, is a valuable time for exchange of ideas and appropriate discussion about patients' emotional and physical needs. Describing the needs of sick people should be accurate, pertinent and without prejudices (Lelean 1973). It is vital to give information about the patients' main concerns or needs. If an opinion is to be expressed the person expressing it should be encouraged 'to own' it, to minimise any opinion that might influence the care of a patient inappropriately. Equally, if nurses are having difficulties managing an aspect of patient care, this can be a good opportunity for the nursing team to solve it through shared discussion and subsequent action.

Medicine rounds

More is learnt about medicines and the function they play in illness if the nurse gives medicines to the patient she is nursing. The procedure of medicine administration is potentially safer if each nurse has fewer patients to whom she gives medicines. She can be encouraged to think of the medicines in relation to her patient's medical condition, symptoms and problems within his activities of living (see Example 5.1). Doctors prescribe using their knowledge base. Nurses who are administering medicines need to be knowledgeable, too, since both

Example 5.1   Giving Patients Medicines

When giving a patient digoxin, the nurse may be asked to think on what she knows about her patient and what observations she is recording. In this way she learns not only what the action of digoxin is, but the reasons why her patient may have:

1. rapid pulse;
2. an apex and radial recording;
3. oedema, feels weak and lethargic;
4. poor skin colour.

This example may be taken a step further when the nurse links medicines she has given with nursing activities such as scoring the patients pressure area risk and observing his oedematous limbs. She can be assisted to make correlations between what she sees and does.

have complementary roles in assessment, efficacy and side-effects of prescribed medicines. The nurse is after all the person who has the most contact with the patients and often has the most up-to-date knowledge of the patient. Two further resources in a hospital are the pharmacist and the drug information bureau. A file containing literature on major drugs makes a useful reference point for nurses and helps when questions are difficult to answer.

Teaching aids on the ward
The inside of the trolley is a good place for visual teaching aids in relation to drugs and their place in certain treatments. Fig. 5.4 illustrates.

Fig. 5.4   Visual aid for medicine trolley

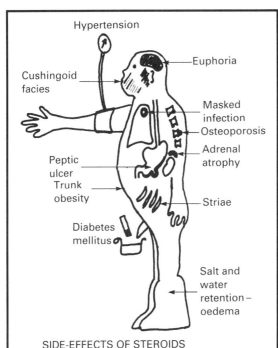

Planning round

The planning round is an opportunity for the registered nurses and student nurse to talk through the care of each patient. The purpose and conduct of planning rounds can differ. Fig. 5.5 gives an example of a set of guidelines that has been used successfully on a general medical ward.

Fig. 5.5   The planning round: guidelines

Aim:
1. To assess, plan and evaluate nursing care under supervision.
2. To discuss and debate issues surrounding the care of individual patients.

Objectives:
1. To assess and plan individualised care with patient or carer, and record this on the care plan.
2. To discuss individual patient problems and their origins relating to medical and nursing management.
3. To demonstrate an awareness of the contribution that members of the multidisciplinary team can make to patient care.
4. To evaluate nursing care by monitoring goal achievements of each patient.
5. To learn how to identify and see priorities in the care of a patient or a group of patients.

The nurse is introduced to her patients by name, having already discussed the patient's relevant biographical details, such as relatives/ friends, occupation and medical diagnosis. The patient may have problems, incapacities and concerns which affect his activities of living. This information, once ascertained, may be recorded under the respective activity of living (for example, eating and drinking). The nurses and students learn from bringing together the knowledge of the patients' incapacities with the patients' data, such as TPR, medicine sheet, etc., as shown in Example 5.2.

Example 5.2   Linking Activities of Living with the Care to be Given

Activity of living	Goal	Care	Linked data
Mr Brown has a sore mouth and throat	to say he can swallow liquids without undue pain	offer cold nutritious drinks with straw. Likes chocolate buildup milk shakes. Clean teeth and corsadyl mouth washes after meals	TPR chart weight medicine sheet (prophylactic drugs; oral candidas)

With the help of good documentation and discussion the nurse can make links between the patients' requirements and professional work. The planning round increases the nurses' knowledge of the patients and helps them and the student put the plan into action and tackle such queries as the following:

- the necessary order of activities;
- which patient needs attention first;
- whether certain procedures or tests are required.

Working together

The novice nurse or student who is new to the ward or the specialty may need advice and guidance on a variety of skills. Skills can be developed by observation and participation as shown in Example 5.3. (The student nurse could equally well be a nurse inexperienced in that procedure.)

Example 5.3   Changing a Dressing

A patient needs a dressing changed around his chest drain site: the student nurse can learn through assisting the registered nurse. The nurse can then go through the following stages with the student nurse:

1. Ask the student nurse what resources she can use for doing this procedure (e.g. as in the nursing procedure book).
2. Suggest she reads the procedure guidelines and/or prepares the trolley for this procedure.
3. Explain precautions needed in this procedure.
4. Describe pneumothorax/haemothorax as relevant.
5. Show an X-ray of the chest.
6. Refer student nurse to: *Manual of Clinical Nursing Procedures*, Royal Marsden Hospital (Pritchard and David (eds.) 1988).
7. Learner observes the registered nurse perform the dressing technique so points previously read or discussed are meaningful and relevant to the patient's safety, comfort and the asepsis of dressing technique. On another occasion, the nurse may observe the student nurse.

Teaching a skill

There are three stages to teaching a skill: explanation; demonstration; and practice. It is important to ensure that there is adequate time for teaching the skill, but that the interval between the stages is not too long (see Fig. 5.6).

Fig. 5.6   Stages in teaching a skill

EXPLANATION	What is the skill, why is it done, how frequently is it done? What is the relationship between theory and practice?
DEMONSTRATION	The teacher demonstrates first at normal speed then more slowly, explaining sequences.
PRACTICE	Time is given for practice under observation. Learner explains what she is doing at each sequence.

In teaching a skill it is helpful to consider the following points:

- During demonstration and practice encourage the nurse to position herself well for observation and comfort so that she is able to concentrate on the skill to be learnt.
- Encourage and acknowledge success achieved.
- Correct mistakes immediately but take care in giving feedback in front of patients so that the patient's confidence in the nurse or student is not destroyed.
- Practice makes perfect, but remember that people vary in dexterity.
- Observations made during a skill performed may need recording in the evaluation section of the care plan because it is a statement of evaluation describing the patient's progress or deterioration; e.g. 'The wound is less red and no longer moist. Patient expresses it is less painful.'
- Suggest the nurse or student consult an article or book on the ward, relating to a recently performed skill.

Learning by observing

The nurse's power of observation is a vital part of successful nursing care. All her senses are involved and much of this kind of information is collected slowly over a period of time and with experience. Nurses may be encouraged to develop 'seeing' skills by showing them *how* to observe and describing *what* they should be looking for. Example 5.4 shows a method for developing observation skills.

Example 5.4   Method for Developing Observation Skills

1. Ask the student nurse to tell you what she sees while giving different patient care. This leads to a dialogue in which the registered nurse fills in the gaps and is able to assess what the student nurse knows, often giving feedback. The patient contributes to this in his personal comments.
2. Talk through a situation that has occurred, recalling what was seen or felt by the nurse and observed in the patient's response to the situation, thus reflecting her nursing care.
3. When care is complete, or a nurse is leaving the patient's room, suggest she looks back and *observes* whether her patient has everything – drink, call bell, looks really comfortable by checking his facial expression or body posture.

Learning through colleagues

Much learning is gained through colleagues; however, nurses do not always become sufficiently involved in discussions with members of the multidisciplinary team. Thus to facilitate learning from the team a number of questions can be considered, such as the following:

- Who are the members of the multidisciplinary team?
- What is the purpose of a multidisciplinary team?
- What are their specialist roles?

It can be helpful to:

- think of two patients and identify what contributions each member is making to the patient in rehabilitation and discharge home,

and then for the 'learner' to perform some of the following:

- Have ten minute exchanges with the physiotherapist, occupational therapist or social worker to either observe their role or their activity with a patient that the nurse/student knows.
- Attend a multidisciplinary team social meeting.
- Plan a discharge in collaboration with members of the team.
- Do a home visit with the occupational therapist.
- Listen to the discussion between a more experienced nurse and physiotherapist.
- Talk to a doctor about his medical plan.

Learning through planning discharges together

Newly registered nurses and students can learn a great deal from discussion and planning of care with a more experienced nurse. This may be concerned with establishing what a patient can do or cannot do as a basis for preparing him for safe discharge. It is important for nurses, together with the members of the multidisciplinary team, to think about their patients achieving appropriate goals in their activities. For example, a patient who lives alone may need to walk between three rooms to wash, dress, eliminate, sleep, cook and eat. These functions are essential for a patient to achieve independently if he lives alone, and he may need practice prior to discharge. Rather like a skill, goal definition needs breaking down into parts so that a nurse may evaluate a patient's capacity to complete his activities of living safely and with confidence.

This process of learning from planning a discharge together can be assisted by the following:

(a) *Defining the goal together:* who will do it, what will be done? Under what circumstances and with what proficiency?
(b) *Observation and participation:* the 'learner' can either observe or participate in a patient referral to the district nurse or health visitor and show her where information files are kept.

Patient education

Preparing patients for discharge often requires nurses to teach a patient new skills or prepare him to adjust to a new experience. For example, the patient may for the first time have to test his urine if he is a newly diagnosed diabetic, or if he is on large doses of steroids, or he may be getting used to a rolator to support his walking.

Nurses know that patient teaching is part of their job but often feel ill-prepared for it. Most patients need help to recover, learn new skills or knowledge to manage illness, incapacities or treatments. Developing an awareness in this aspect of nursing care is vital and the responsibility for patient education is usually shared between doctors and nurses. Observing a more experienced nurse when involved in teaching her patients can be beneficial. There are also articles to read (for example, as brought together in the book *Patient Education Plus*, by The Professional Nurse, 1990) and Health Education Authority leaflets that are available for patients.

One useful way of encouraging nurses to increase their skills in patient education is for them to be involved in a small 'project' related to the ward; for example the development of a booklet/leaflet on what to expect after surgery, the preparation of information for patients who are about to be discharged home, to help them in the management of their diabetes or in coping with a bronchial disorder.

Learning from specialist nurses

There is an increasing use of nurses for specialist areas of care; for example oncology, care of the dying, diabetic liaison and stoma therapy. Registered nurses and students can learn a great deal from such nurses, both by the referral and discussion of the care of particular patients, and by inviting specialist nurses to the ward to talk about their role.

Formal teaching and learning opportunities

A planned programme of topics

Formal teaching has a place in each ward provided it is planned, relevant and well publicised. The nursing team should plan it together so that it reflects the team's own needs and acts as useful input for students. Topics can be wide ranging, including how the nursing care is organised, specific aspects of care, opportunities for professional development, use of research on the ward, and so on. Other personnel may be involved such as doctors, pharmacist, chaplain, dietitian. Some examples of topics are as follows:

- *General*, e.g. implications of Project 2000; implications of the White Paper at ward level; ethical considerations.
- *Management*, e.g. primary nursing; health and safety; disciplinary action.
- *Research*, e.g. research on mouth care; communication.
- *Clinical*, e.g. care of a patient with specific problems; technical skill such as learning about suction equipment.

Discussions related to events

Discussions about problems and events are semi-formal learning opportunities. Short discussions are valuable if proper time is set aside and the discussion responds to staff needs. Those involved should be the participants in an event, and the discussion should be held near the time that the event occurred.

Discussions are facilitated by: a comfortable location; time set aside; the appointment of a leader to convene the group and get it started but not to dominate it; encouragement to analyse and learn from the event, not just to describe it; a summary of the conclusions and/or action.

Examples of possible situations to explore are as follows:

- a fire in the kitchen;
- a patient complains about a member of staff;

- ethical dilemma such as a patient who is unable to eat but is very incapacitated by a stroke;
- a patient who is difficult to cope with and is becoming increasingly unpopular;
- nurses consistently going off duty late;
- a young patient who has recently died and the staff are feeling sad;
- drug error.

A great deal can be learnt from the analysis of problems and events. For example: consider how they arose, what action was taken, whether the outcome was satisfactory, whether improvements could be made.

Presenting a patient care plan
Each nurse can be given a formal opportunity to present a patient she has nursed to a group of colleagues. This can help individuals to develop skills and confidence in preparing material and talking to a group. The speaker discusses a patient she has nursed with specific reference to his nursing care, problems encountered, what could have been improved and what she has learnt.

Critically discussing a journal article
One way of encouraging nurses to read journals, and make use of the knowledge that is gained, is for nurses to be asked to choose an article from a nursing journal, summarise its contents, outline its implications for nursing care – and then present it to a group of nurses and learners in such a way that others too, might, learn from the main points.

Alerting others to learning opportunities
Posters can be displayed – using colours and large print – which list the learning opportunities on the ward and the unit. Example 5.5 illustrates one in use on a medical ward; it would, however, be relevant for many clinical settings. In addition, teaching can be logged in a ward book. This not only helps with the organisation of ward teaching and future ward learning audits, but it also helps ward staff to value retrospective work.

Literature and information
Box files can be very useful for storing references. Examples include:

- assessment guidelines for each activity of living (Roper *et al.* 1986);
- the students' aims and objectives pertaining to the ward experience;
- learning contracts of registered nurses if these are not personal, confidential documents;
- research literature relevant to current nursing activity.

Example 5.5   Opportunities for Learning on the Ward: A Ward Poster
(adapted from an original by Janice Sigsworth)

There are many ways in which nurses and students can learn more on this ward. These are just some of the opportunities available for you:

1. Monthly journals (e.g. *Professional Nurse and Senior Nurse*)
2. Filing cabinet full of articles – please add new ones that you find helpful
3. Special subject folders (book shelf)
4. Notice board
5. Weekly lectures or seminars
6. Student meetings
7. Planning rounds
8. Ward objectives
9. Working with a registered nurse; assessing, planning, giving and evaluating care
10. Self-assessment (for students)
11. Peer review (for registered nurses)

Conclusion

The process of nurse learning is influenced by the opportunities and experiences that the nurse or student has in the settings in which she nurses patients and relates to a multidisciplinary team. The registered nurse is a key person in determining how and what students learn and in trying to ensure that theory is related to practice. There are many ways in which learning can be facilitated or minimised. At the heart, however, is the fact that nurses are adult learners; they thrive on seeing and experiencing rather than simply on being told. This is reflected in the old Chinese proverb:

> I hear and I forget
> I see and I remember

The whole role and status of those learning to nurse is changing with Project 2000 which in turn will affect the newly registered nurse's teaching responsibilities. Some will find the new expectations of them as mentors quite difficult, particularly where they are struggling to learn so many new things themselves. Others will rise to the challenge and accept that passing on their knowledge to others, and helping others to learn as much as possible is a normal and fulfilling part of their job. This chapter has tried to provide some practical ways to achieve good teaching and effective learning.

References

Argyris, C. and Schön, D. A. (1974) *Theory in Practice: Increasing Professiona Effectiveness*, San Francisco: Jossey Bass.

Atkins, S. (1990) *Preparing to Mentor Undergraduates – Nurses' Expressed Needs* Unpublished Research Study, Department of Health Care Studies, Oxforc Polytechnic.

Ausubel, D. (1978) *Educational Psychology: A Cognitive View*, New York: Holt Rinehart and Winston.

Bandura, A. (1977) *Social Learning Theory*, New Jersey: Prentice Hall.

Benner, P. (1984) *From Novice to Expert: Excellence and Power in Clinical Nursin Practice*, California: Addison Wesley.

Boud, D., Keogh, R. and Walker, D. (1985) *Reflection: Turning Experience intc Learning*, London: Kogan Page.

Bracken, E. and Davis, J. (1989) 'The implications of mentorship in nursing caree development', *Senior Nurse*, Vol. 9, No. 5, pp. 15–6.

Bradshaw, P. (ed.) (1989) *Teaching and Assessing in Clinical Nursing Practice*, Heme Hempstead: Prentice Hall.

Burnard, P. (1988) 'A supporting act', *Nursing Times*, Vol. 84, No. 46, pp. 27–8.

Daloz, L. A. (1986) *Effective Teaching and Mentoring*, San Francisco: Jossey Bass.

Darbyshire, P., Stewart, B., Jamieson, L. and Tongue, C. (1990) 'New domains ir nursing', *Nursing Times*, Vol. 86, No. 27, pp. 73–5.

Darling, L. A. W. (1984) 'What do nurses want in a mentor?' *The Journal of Nursing Administration*, Vol. 14, No. 10, pp. 42–4.

Donovan, J. (1990) 'The concept and role of mentor', *Nurse Education Today*, Vol. 10 pp. 294–8.

ENB Circular 1987/28/MAT *Institutional and Course Approval/Reapproval Process, Information Required, Criteria and Guidelines*, London: English National Board.

ENB (1987) *Managing Change in Nursing Education*, London: English Nationa Board.

ENB Circular 1988/39/APS *Institutional and Course Approval/Reapproval Process, Information Required, Criteria and Guidelines*, London: English National Board.

Farnish, S. (1983) *Ward Sister Preparation: A Survey in Three Districts*, Chelsea College: University of London.

Fretwell, J. (1980) 'An inquiry into the ward learning environment', *Nursing Times Occasional Paper*, Vol. 76, No. 16, pp. 69–75.

Fretwell, J. (1982) *Ward Teaching and Learning*, London: Royal College o Nursing.

George, P. (1987) *The Nurse as a Reflective Practitioner*, Unpublished Paper, Oxforc Polytechnic.

Hilgard, R. E. and Atkinson, R. C. (1967) *Introduction to Psychology*, 4th edn, New York: Harcourt Brace Jovanovich.

Jacka, K. and Lewin, D. (1987) *The Clinical Learning of Student Nurses*, Kings College University of London.

Jarvis, P. (1983) *Professional Education*, London: Croom Helm.

Jarvis, P. and Gibson, S. (1985) *The Teacher Practitioner in Nursing Midwifery and Health Visiting*, London: Croom Helm.

Jarvis, P. (1986) 'Contract learning', *Journal of District Nursing*, November, pp. 13–14.

Kenworthy, N. and Nicklin, P. (1989) *Teaching and Assessing in Nursing Practice: An Experiential Approach*, London: Scutari Press.

Knowles, M. (1970) *The Modern Practice of Adult Education: Andragogy Versus Pedagogy*, Chicago: Follett.

Knowles, M. (1984) *Andragogy in Action: Applying Modern Principles of Adult Education*, San Francisco: Jossey Bass.

Kolb, D. A. and Fry, R. (1975) 'Towards an applied theory of experiential learning', in Cooper, G. L. (ed.) *Theories of Group Processes*, Chichester: John Wiley and Sons.

Kolb, D. A. (1984) *Experiential Learning*, New Jersey: Prentice Hall.

Lathlean, J., Smith, G. and Bradley, S. (1986) *Post-Registration Development Schemes Evaluation*, Kings College, University of London.

Lathlean, J. and Vaughan, B. (eds.) (in press) *Bridging the Gap: Unifying nursing practice and theory*, London: Harper Collins.

Lee, H. (1989) 'Them and us: closing the gap between theory and practice', *Senior Nurse*, Vol. 9, No. 8, pp. 17–19.

Lelean, S. (1973) *Ready for Report, Nurse?* London: Royal College of Nursing.

MacLeod, M. L. P. (1990) *Experience in Everyday Nursing Practice: A Study of 'Experienced' Surgical Ward Sisters.* Unpublished PhD Thesis, University of Edinburgh.

Major, S. (1989) 'Teaching and learning: a climate of change', *Nursing Standard*, Vol. 4, No. 3, pp. 36–8.

Marson, S. (1981) *Ward Teaching Skills – an Investigation into the Behavioural Characteristics of Effective Ward Teachers.* Unpublished MPhil Thesis, Sheffield City Polytechnic.

Maslow, A. (1970) *Motivation and Personality*, 2nd edn, New York: Harper and Row.

May, K. (1982) 'Mentorship for scholarliness', *Nursing Outlook*, Vol. 30, pp. 22–6.

McEvoy, P. (1989) 'A new model for learning', *Senior Nurse*, Vol. 9, No. 2, pp. 27–9.

Miles, R. (1987) 'Experiential learning in the curriculum', in Allan, P. and Jolley, M. (eds.) *The Curriculum in Nursing Education*, Beckenham: Croom Helm.

Moore, D. J. (1989) 'Four approaches to teaching and learning', in Bradshaw, P. (ed.) *Teaching and Assessing in Clinical Nursing Practice*, Hemel Hempstead: Prentice Hall.

Morle, K. (1990) 'Mentorship – is it the case of the emperor's new clothes or a rose by any other name?' *Nurse Education Today*, Vol. 10, No. 1, pp. 66–9.

Morris, N., John, G. and Keen, T. (1988) 'Learning the ropes', *Nursing Times*, Vol. 84, No. 46.

Norton, E. (1989) 'Contract learning in nurse education: bridging the theory/practice gap', *Senior Nurse*, Vol. 9, No. 8, pp. 21–3.

Ogier, M. (1982) *An Ideal Sister? A Study of the Leadership Style and Verbal Interactions of Ward Sisters with Nurse Learners in General Hospitals*, London: Royal College of Nursing.

Ogier, M. (1989) *Working and Learning*, London: Scutari Press.

Orton, H. D. (1981) *Ward Learning Climate: A Study of the Role of the Ward Sister in Relation to Student Nurse Learning on the Ward*, London: Royal College of Nursing.

Pavlov, I. P. (1960) *Conditioned Reflexes*, New York: Dover (a reprint of Pavlov, I. P. (1927) *Conditioned Reflexes* (trans. by G. V. Anrep) London: Oxford).

Pembrey, S. E. M. (1980) *The Ward Sister – Key to Nursing*, London: Royal College of Nursing.

Powell, J. H. (1989) 'The reflective practitioner in nursing', *Journal of Advanced Nursing*, Vol. 14, pp. 824–32.

Quinn, F. M. (1988) *The Principles and Practice of Nurse Education*, London: Croom Helm.

Reid, N. G. (1986) *Wards in Chancery?* London: Royal College of Nursing.

Rogers, C. (1969) *Freedom to Learn*, Columbus, Ohio: C. E. Merril.

Rogers, C. (1983) *Freedom to Learn for the 80s*, Columbus, Ohio: C. E. Merril.

Roper, N., Logan, W. and Tierney, A. (1983) *Using a Model for Nursing*, Edinburgh: Churchill-Livingstone.

Schön, D. A. (1983) *The Reflective Practitioner: How Professionals Think in Action*, New York: Basic Books.

Sigsworth, J. and Heslop, A. (1988) 'Self-assessment and the student nurse', *Senior Nurse*, Vol. 8, No. 5.

Skelton, G. M. (1989) 'Assessment and profiling of clinical performance', in Bradshaw, P. (ed.) *Teaching and Assessing in Clinical Nursing Practice*, Hemel Hempstead: Prentice Hall.

Skinner, B. F. (1953) *Science and Human Behaviour*, New York: Macmillan.

Talarczyk, K. and Milbrandt, D. (1988) 'A collaborative effort to facilitate role transition from student to registered nurse practitioner', *Nursing Management*, Vol. 19, No. 2, pp. 30–2.

The Professional Nurse (1990) *Patient Education Plus*, London: Austen Cornish Publishers.

Thorndike, E. L. (1928) *Adult Learning*, London: Macmillan.

United Kingdom Central Council (1987) *Project 2000: The Final Proposals*, Project Paper 9, London: UKCC.

United Kingdom Central Council for Nursing, Midwifery and Health Visiting (1990) *The Report of the Post-Registration Education and Practice Project (PREPP)*, London: UKCC.

Wright, S. (1986) *Building and Using a Model of Nursing*, London: Edward Arnold.

Wright, S. (1989) 'Supporting learners in the workplace', in Robinson, K. (ed.) *Open and Distance Learning for Nurses*, Harlow: Longman.

6   Stress

INGRID STEVENS

Introduction

The transition from student to staff nurse has been identified as a difficult phase of development in that many newly registered nurses perceive their roles as stressful (Vaughan 1980, Lathlean *et al.* 1986). Various factors give rise to feelings of stress in individuals, and work has been undertaken on the meaning or concept of stress, and ways of coping with, or alleviating it. A central focus of this work is the need to recognise stress in oneself and, in turn, in others, and there are various practical ways of doing this. However, there is no simple formula available for dealing with stress – each person will perceive and cope with it differently and it is important to realise the individuality of the notion of stress. Neither is stress always dysfunctional, and a certain level of pressure for some people is helpful.

Stress and the newly registered nurse

Lathlean *et al.* (1986) identified stresses experienced by individual newly registered nurses (see Fig. 6.1). They point out that, of the nurses studied, it was not only the vulnerable individuals who suffered stress. Their findings indicate that the causes of stress also went beyond the individual, and that newly registered nurses perceive stress differently. Consequently, the examples given were not perceived as stressful by all of the group.

Newly registered nurses found being in charge of a ward stressful. Lack of recognition by other staff of their new status and inexperience was identified as being one aspect of this, a finding confirmed in another research study of staff nurses conducted by Binnie (1988). The sudden role change with marked increase in responsibility and perceived inadequate preparation and support was also found to contribute to the stress. For example, Lathlean *et al.* (1986) identified recently qualified nurses who were concerned about 'something going wrong', and 'having to stand up and be counted' and Binnie's (1988) study

Fig. 6.1   Stresses experienced by newly registered nurses (Source:
Lathlean *et al.* 1986)

Being in charge of the ward
Responsibility for patients, learners and self
Difficulties establishing authority
Multiple demands upon nurse in charge
Difficult relationships with medical staff
Communication with the patients' relatives
Caring for dying patients
Inadequacy to support learners
Lack of NRN role definition
Lack of support and feedback
Lack of opportunities for self-development
Inadequate standards of care

included a respondent who typically 'felt an awful lot of responsibility and used to go home and not sleep, or dream about booking transport'. The diversity of responsibilities and the feeling of inability to cope with a myriad of tasks was a feature of both the above-mentioned research studies.

Being the focal point of information on the ward was stressful, compounded by the nurse's difficulties communicating with medical staff and patients' relatives. Relationships with medical staff were not always found to be easy when the new nurse was in charge of the ward, during ward rounds, and when she handled criticism which she thought to be unfair. It seems, though, that this is not only a problem for the newly registered nurse, as illustrated by a nurse who had been qualified for some time: 'I know when things are going wrong and would like a patient to be seen by doctors, and they don't listen to you . . . they obviously don't hold you in very high esteem.' (Binnie 1988).

Relationships with dying patients and their relatives were found to be stressful, particularly if death occurred unexpectedly. Breaking the news of death, supporting bereaved relatives and caring for dying patients of a similar age to the nurse were especially difficult, and more so if the nurse herself was recently bereaved. Newly registered nurses felt inadequate in caring for dying patients, saying that talking to the patient about his or her prognosis was particularly problematic. These difficulties are examples of activities which many of the nurses had not undertaken before, and the stress of learning new tasks was emphasised.

Few clinical aspects were found to be stressful except caring for confused and demanding patients (as defined by the nurses themselves), dealing with cardiac arrests and caring for a high proportion of very ill or chronically sick patients. Nurses in Binnie's (1988) study sometimes found technical aspects of their job threatening, such as the use of monitors. A further cause of stress for the new nurse was lack of clarity regarding her role, sudden changes in role (e.g. being in charge of the ward intermittently), and decreased patient contact.

The ward itself and the organisation of the ward work can also be a source of stress, for example through low standards of care, inadequate staffing, heavy workload, working without meal breaks, and lack of continuity of staff. The need to undertake non-nursing duties, and the lack of administrative help such as a ward clerk were identified as contributing factors. Frequent absence of ward sisters causing lack of support and leadership, poor inter-staff communication and lack of peer support were also highlighted. Newly registered nurses felt the need for feedback regarding their performance, positive reinforcement, reassurance and knowledge that others were struggling too. They required an opportunity to discuss their difficulties with others, particularly their peers.

It appears that stress changes over time, often with a progressive increase during the first three months, followed by a reduction by the end of six months, with fluctuations and subsequent peaks due to specific events. This is illustrated in Fig. 6.2.

Fig. 6.2   The change in stress over time (After Binnie 1988)

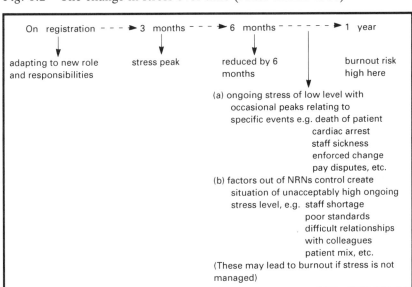

The nature of stress

Individual perceptions of stress, and of self, are key factors which influence how individual nurses cope with stress. Stress is defined as 'a perceptual imbalance between demand and capability' (Gillespie and Gillespie 1986). Each individual has her own view of the demands upon herself. Stress occurs when the individual perceives that she is incapable of handling the demands.

Why does demand exceed a newly qualified nurse's capability? A pilot study undertaken by the author indicated that experienced registered nurses, and newly qualified nurses in an unfamiliar specialty, commonly doubt their own ability to meet demands made upon them. For example, a staff nurse new to oncology nursing, although registered for twenty-two months, described informing a spouse that her husband's condition had deteriorated: 'I rang his wife, which I'd not really done before . . . I was concerned that there was nobody with her. I didn't know if I was going about it in quite the right way. She'd got a three quarters of an hour drive – in about 10 minutes he'd died.'

This is a common situation. The stress here appears to be due to the staff nurse's *perception* that she may lack the experience and skills to meet the needs of the wife effectively. The nurse doubted her own abilities, and this doubt is an internal demand causing her stress. Simultaneously, the staff nurse had other, external demands to consider. She said: 'I felt bad that we hadn't realised how ill he was earlier, because we had another patient on the ward who needed the attention of all nurses on the shift. I kept going back to him, and he looked asleep.' These external demands involved the staff nurse managing the ward for that shift, and re-allocating staff due to the unexpected changes in both these patients.

This example illustrates the view that 'demand is an internal or external stimulus which is perceived by the individual as requiring an adaptive response' (Clarke 1984). An adaptive *response* is how that nurse responds to all the demands made upon her. Which demands did she respond to first, and why? How did she respond? She defined her priorities. First, she appears to have met the safety needs of both patients by re-allocation of staff. Then she telephoned the wife of the patient who was deteriorating. This is how she coped. *Coping* has been described as 'a response carried out by the individual and appraised by him, as either satisfactorily or unsatisfactorily affecting the demand in the desired direction' (Clarke 1984). The staff nurse maintained the safety of both patients, but did not meet the needs of the wife to her (the staff nurse's) satisfaction.

The staff nurse appraised the effectiveness of her coping as follows: 'I don't feel unduly stressed by it, I just don't feel satisfied by it. There were certain things that were beyond my control. I just feel I'd like to have done more. I don't think I do cope actually. I think that experience probably helps.' Her *appraisal* indicates that her coping efforts affected the demands but not all demands achieved the desired direction. She is left with mixed feelings, and she identifies the influence of control. Failure to recognise the limitations of the situation and of herself could have resulted in higher stress and a poorer appraisal of her coping efforts.

Threats are perceived differently according to circumstances. Folkman *et al.* (1986) suggest that the individual and the context shape coping efforts. Coping depends upon the individual, the context and the demand itself. If the demand is perceived to cause harm or loss it is a threat. If the demand can be mastered it is a challenge. A staff nurse, eleven months into her first post, describes a threat. She feels unable to master the demands upon her. She described the situation: 'It was that particular evening and her attitude towards me . . . I found annoying. I'm quite intimidated by students generally because of the implied capability that you are supposed to have, and I don't feel capable most of the time, I'll admit. And her attitude, it was far more blatant than many, and it really rammed it home that I find the students threatening' (Stevens 1989).

Coping involves appraisal. Alternative coping efforts may be evaluated before a strategy is chosen. The staff nurse perceived her alternatives as: 'I can try to avoid it (the problem = student nurse) or 'I can confront it' by taking the student aside and counselling her. She took the former alternative. The coping strategy used involved emotional, cognitive and behavioural elements. Anger was felt initially as described above. Later coping involved specific behaviour and analysis. As she said: 'I smoked, drank, and talked to a friend, to work out why I did what I did, and how I did it.' The processes that this staff nurse followed can be illustrated by a flow chart as shown in Fig. 6.3.

Coping strategies employed by different people vary and they include some or all of the following:

● escape, e.g. distraction, avoidance;
● methods of tension reduction, e.g. non-competitive exercise, massage;
● seeking support and information, e.g. self-help groups, talking to colleagues and friends;
● setting realistic expectations of self/role;
● acceptance of self.

Strategies are individual or collective and can be divided into the following three types:

1. *Direct coping*: requires the nurse to tackle the cause of the stress, e.g. confronting the problem by taking action to change it.
2. *Indirect coping*: helps the nurse develop techniques to manage stress, e.g. relaxation, distraction.
3. *Palliative coping*: makes the coper feel better without dealing with the cause of the stress, e.g. eating, smoking, drinking alcohol.

The purpose of coping, according to Bailey (1985), is to achieve homeostatic functioning (or stability) as shown in Fig. 6.4.

The subject of coping in nursing is tackled well by Clarke (1989) and further guidance can be gained by referring to this book.

Fig. 6.3   Flow chart: the processes of coping (Source: Stevens 1989)

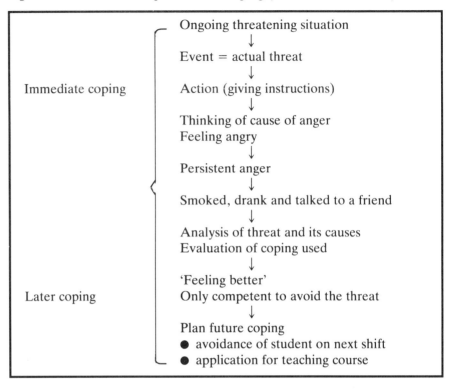

Fig. 6.4   The purpose of coping (Source: Bailey 1985)

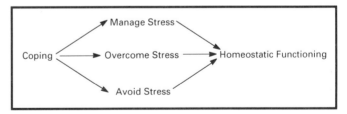

The value of stress

It is important to remember that stress is not entirely negative or destructive. Total lack of stress is detrimental to health. Arousal is necessary, and sufficient stimulation is required to promote optimum functioning (Atkinson *et al.* 1983). The ideal, therefore, is a balance between overstimulation by excessive demands, and understimulation by lack of demands. Equilibrium is achieved when capability matches demand (see Fig. 6.5).

Fig. 6.5   The balance between over-and under stimulation

OVER STIMULATION	UNDER STIMULATION
Effects upon individual	*Effects upon individual*
Anxiety	Fatigue
Stress	Boredom
Lack of satisfaction	Lack of satisfaction

   Castledine (1988) suggests that 'stress from positive challenges which promote, even demand, individual growth and achievement are desirable and are good stress'. Mastering a stressful challenge can promote personal growth. Hingley (1984) points out that people do recognise and appreciate positive aspects of stress. He supports Castledine's view, suggesting that stress gets work done, improves efficiency and can be an effective monitor. However, Bamber (1988) emphasises the harmful nature of stress over a long period of time. Further, he observes that nurses' occupational stress is linked with stress in their private lives and concludes that even mild stress can result in drug taking, overuse of alcohol and lead to people dropping out from the profession. It is clear, then, that mild signs of stress must not be ignored and allowed to develop, rendering the individual at risk of potentially life-threatening or impairing forms of palliative coping.

The effects of unrecognised and unalleviated stress

Recognition of stress requires understanding of stress processes, their causes and manifestations. Bailey (1985) suggests that 'caring can damage your health' in that stress is now accepted as being a hazard for those in the caring professions; indeed, doctors, nurses and other carers are at greater risk of stress problems than the general population. Hingley (1984) also finds evidence of the effects of stress, citing nursing as a profession with one of the highest rates of suicide as well as nurses topping the list of psychiatric outpatient referrals. Hingley suggests that little is known about the degree, extent, causes, effects and ways of relieving stress.

   It seems advisable to consider how stress can be identified in order to be able to prevent or relieve it. Bailey (1985) offers some criteria that may be of value (see Fig. 6.6). The questions in Fig. 6.6 can be tried out during a stressful time, e.g. prior to major examinations or an important interview. Fig. 6.7 identifies some of the signs to look for and Cox (1985) provides a comprehensive list of the effects of stress (Fig. 6.8).

Fig. 6.6 Recognition of stress process in an individual (Source: Bailey 1985)

1. Is there a loss of psychological functioning compared with previously?
2. Is there a loss of physical functioning compared with previously?
3. Is there a psychological/physical loss of health over a period of time?
4. What coping efforts has the person used to overcome, ameliorate or avoid circumstances?
5. Are these coping efforts helpful or counterproductive?

Fig. 6.7 Signs of mild stress (Source: Bamber 1988)

- Recent lack of enjoyment of life generally
- Increase in weight
- Smoking too much
- Increased heart rate
- Dry mouth
- Indigestion
- Depression
- Anxiety

Fig. 6.8 Health effects suggested to be linked to stress (Source: Cox 1985)

Subjective effects
Anxiety, aggression, apathy, boredom, depression, fatigue, frustration, guilt and shame, irritability and bad temper, moodiness, low self-esteem, threat and tension, nervousness and loneliness.

Behavioural effects
Accident proneness, drug taking, emotional outbursts, excessive eating or loss of appetite, excessive drinking and smoking, excitability, impulsive behaviour, impaired speech, nervous laughter, restlessness, trembling.

Cognitive effects
Inability to make decisions and concentrate, frequent forgetfulness, hypersensitivity to criticism, mental blocks.

Physiological effects
Increased blood and urine catecholamines and corticosteroids, increased blood glucose levels, increased heart rate and blood pressure, dryness of mouth, sweating, dilation of pupils, difficulty breathing, hot and cold spells, a lump in the throat, numbness and tingling in parts of the limbs.

Health effects
Asthma, amenorrhoea, chest and back pains, coronary heart disease, diarrhoea, faintness and dizziness, dyspepsia, frequent urination, headaches and migraine, neuroses, nightmares, psychoses, psycho-somatic disorders, diabetes mellitus, skin rash, ulcers, loss of sexual interest and weakness.

Organisational effects
Absenteeism, poor industrial relations, poor productivity, high accident and labour turnover, poor organisational climate, antagonism at work and job dissatisfaction.

Recognition of the effects of stress is an important part of managing it. Their relevance to stress management is whether these symptoms of stress are temporary, recurring or long-term and whether they are acute or chronic. The stress process is progressive, and negative effects need to be monitored. Long-term implications of stress include coronary heart disease and alcohol abuse. Examples of acute responses to stress in newly qualified nurses include feeling scared, angry, inadequate, shaky, upset and wanting to leave nursing, feeling overburdened, and feeling terrified, unsupported, stressed and worrying for ages afterwards (Humphries 1987).

One of the ways of identifying stress, as a first step towards its management, is to reflect on one's own feelings and reactions. Exercise 6.1, whilst relatively simple, can aid the process of identifying stress in self and in others.

Exercise 6.1   Identifying stress in yourself and others

How does stress affect you personally? Consider how you feel when you are stressed. Think of 3 stressful situations in which you have been involved.

1. What were your signs of stress (a) immediately? (b) later?
2. How did you cope (a) immediately? (b) later?
3. What did you learn from this experience?

Now consider your colleagues in these situations. Focus on one of them. What were his/her signs of stress? How did he/she cope?

Burnout

If stress remains unrecognised and unalleviated, burnout is likely to occur eventually. Burnout is a response to excessive stress and is itself a progressive stress process. Definitions vary but there is general consensus that 'burnout is characterised by a pronounced stress state over time' (Bailey 1985). Burnout is, therefore, a process involving changing symptoms: 'a syndrome of emotional exhaustion, involving the development of negative self-concept, negative job attitudes, and loss of crucial concern and feelings for clients' (Maslach in Bailey 1985) – see Fig. 6.9.

Fig. 6.9   The process of burnout (Source: Bailey 1985)

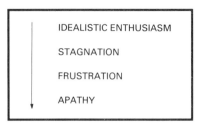

Bailey (1985) suggests that there are three main stages in this burnout process, and describes symptoms which may occur (see Fig. 6.10).

Fig. 6.10   Phases in the burnout process (Source: Bailey 1985)

Phase 1: Physical symptoms
Exhaustion, fatigue, lingering colds, headaches, gastro-intestinal disturbances, sleeplessness, breathlessness, skin complaints, general aches and pains.

Phase 2: Psychological, behavioural and social symptoms
Irritability, unprovoked angry outbursts, easily moved to tears, marked sadness, screaming and shouting, unwarranted suspicion and paranoia, lethargy, avoiding commitment to caring.
Relationships with people decreasing in importance, negative feelings about work, impaired mental abilities, e.g. impaired problem-solving and listening.
Withdrawal from clients and colleagues, increased consumption of alcohol, drugs and cigarettes.

Phase 3: Final phase
Guilt about negative feelings and behaviour, anger at self, depression, feeling a total failure.

The symptoms include those of stress but with the following differences:

● sheer exhaustion;
● the unpredictable nature of phase 2; and

● the entirely negative and introverted nature of phase 3.

Recognition of symptoms in oneself and in colleagues is important if the burnout process is to be stopped. Following a checklist can be helpful – whether it is a memorised list of symptoms or a specially designed tool such as Bailey's Burnout Checklist (see Fig. 6.11).

Often an individual who is passing through the phases of burnout may not realise it unless she takes the time to review not only her work performance, but her life style generally and her physical and mental health. Undertaking a regular review, say once a month or every two months, using the same checklist, can be a helpful means of comparison over a period.

Thus recognition can involve the following:

● a mental or written checklist;
● comparison with previous checklists;
● re-reading a diary and identifying risk factors and symptoms;
● discussions with colleagues and friends about personal and professional life;
● taking part in a formalised support group with focused discussion.

Causes of burnout

McElroy (1982) suggests that causes of burnout in oncology nurses are internal and external, multiple and occur progressively. She categorises the causes as social, personal, educational, professional and institutional (see Fig. 6.12). McElroy's evidence, upon which she bases this list, is tenuous – often anecdotal. However, if it provokes questioning and reflective thoughts in the reader, it is worthy of consideration. Many of the causes identified appear to be part of the nurse's work and environment. Solutions to burnout must, therefore, extend beyond the individual. On the other hand, some causes are specifically related to each individual, the most obvious being personality. Freudenberger (1974) argues that personality is an important influence. Individuals identified as being at high risk of burnout tend to be dedicated and overcommitted; they substitute work for social life; they are authoritarian; they view themselves as indispensible; and they overidentify with clients. These ideas are neither proven or disproved; they merit consideration but in conjunction with other factors.

Hingley and Harris (1986) believe stress awareness in the profession to be low. They argue that stress is not seen as a solvable problem, the prevailing attitude appearing to be that 'nurses should either put up with the difficulties or get out . . . a painful reminder that intolerance and lack of understanding about nurses' stress and burnout still occurs in this so-called caring profession.'

Fig. 6.11   Burnout inventory (Source: Bailey 1985)

Burn-Out Inventory

This is a Burn-out Inventory which may be completed by setting up a Burn-out checklist similar to the example on the facing page. On your checklist simply make a check against each item which applies to you. A number of stress-checks may be carried out (e.g. before, during and after practising stress control). By doing this you could compare the items you have checked on the Burn-out Checklist with the practice of stress-control training. You may wish to keep a separate note of any changes that have taken place and benefits which you have observed.

Procedure

1. Draw up your own Burn-out Checklist and on it make a check mark against any item as it applies to you at present.
2. Add up the number of items you have checked, e.g. 10 burn-out items.
3. Select an appropriate stress-control technique and put it into practice.
4. Practise stress control for a specific number of weeks (e.g. 1, 4, 6, 10, etc.)
5. After completing each practice period, reassess yourself on your Burn-out Inventory.
6. Now make any comparisons with your previous assessment.
7. If you are satisfied, you may stop stress-control training. But if you want to, continue with the same stress-control training or other stress-control procedures.
8. Repeat any reassessment and further stress-control training if necessary.

Note: You may find it helpful to discuss items on your Burn-out Inventory and stress-control training programme with your collegues, tutor-advisor or counsellor.

Fig. 6.11   (contd)

Burn-Out Checklist	Assessment				
	1	2	3	4	5
1. High resistance to going to work every day.					
2. A sense of failure.					
3. Anger and resentment.					
4. Guilt and blame.					
5. Discouragement and indifference.					
6. Negativism.					
7. Isolation and withdrawal.					
8. Feeling tired and exhausted all day.					
9. Frequent clockwatching.					
10. Great fatigue after work.					
11. Loss of positive feelings towards clients/patients.					
12. Postponing client contacts; resisting client phone calls and office visits.					
13. Stereotyping clients.					
14. Inability to concentrate or listen to what clients or colleagues are saying.					
15. Feeling immobilized.					
16. Cynicism regarding clients-colleagues; a blaming attitude.					
17. Increasingly 'going by the book'.					
18. Sleep disorders.					
19. Avoiding discussion of work with colleagues.					
20. Self-preoccupation.					
21. More approving of behaviour-control measures such as tranquillizers.					
22. Frequent colds and flus.					
23. Frequent headaches.					
24. Rigidity in thinking and resistance to change.					
25. Suspicion and paranoia.					
26. Excessive use of drugs e.g. alcohol, tobacco products, etc.					
27. Marital and family conflict.					
28. High absenteeism.					
29. Skin complaints, e.g. rashes etc.					
30. Gastrointestinal disturbances.					
Number of symptoms					

Fig. 6.12   Causes of burnout in oncology nurses (Source: McElroy 1982)

Social causes
Individual's needs for 'self-actualisation'.
Individual's needs for competence and success.
Responsibility for the well-being of others in the health care services.
Population mobility and lack of family and community ties.

Personal causes
Personality types.
Unrealistically high standards of care.
Strong need to be accepted and liked.

Educational causes
Highly idealistic nurse.
Belief that there is a resolution to every problem.

Professional causes
Nursing specialities may have different burnout risks.
Physical setting.
Difficult decision making and working under pressure can undermine nurse's energy and coping ability.
Communication difficulties between nurses and doctors.

Institutional causes
'The source of burnout lies more in situations than people'.
Large organisations – tendency to absenteeism, turnover, job dissatisfaction.
Bureaucratic red tape.
Lack of meaningful leadership.
Inadequate communication.
Impaired supervision.
Narrowly defined job descriptions.
Professional conflicts, e.g. role overload, ideal versus real, role ambiguity.

Management of stress in self and others

At an individual level, stress management focuses upon an individual's coping strategies and their effectiveness. An important factor underpinning these strategies is the individual's philosophy of nursing and of life. Newlin and Wellisch (1978) advocate a professional philosophy for oncology nurses whereby the nurse gains rewards from providing comfort to the patient and emotional support to the patient and family. This emphasises the value of comfort and support, and the skills required to achieve them. Formal recognition of these values provides clarity of purpose, and raises self-esteem when the goals have been achieved. Eliezer (1981) suggests that a philosophy of life helps in oncology nursing and argues that 'the way to look at life, self, giving, and living has a personal supportive role in the day to day caring for people with cancer'.

It seems reasonable to think that a philosophy of life could be helpful to all nurses in all specialities. Bamber (1988) suggests that the nurse should not be afraid to say 'this is only a job for which I get paid', and 'I am the most important person I know'. Beliefs and values such as these are likely to influence perception of self and role, colleagues and situations. A study of Nichols *et al.* (1981) indicates that registered nurses working in ITU felt stressed when their autonomy was not recognised and the nurses perceived their status to be low. His findings suggest that there is a link between perceiving stress and self-esteem.

Stress can be managed in the following ways:

- *Clear definition of role*, and confidence to take on that role, can promote a positive perspective. Consequently, the nurse is more likely to perceive demands as challenges than as stresses. Drawing up a job description with a senior nurse, and identifying the post-holder's specific responsibilities, is essential for every nurse prior to accepting a post. This is one way of minimising work stress and promoting job satisfaction. Designated responsibility can be constructive, leading to motivation, realistic ambition, and a sense of achievement.
- *Reflecting* about oneself and one's actions is a useful starting point when trying both to understand stresses and to develop. Writing a diary can be a good means of reflecting upon physical and psychological well-being. Reading back over the diary subsequently can provide insight into feelings and behaviour.
- *Group discussions* about the nature of the work, about personal difficulties and strengths can be a way of identifying symptoms of stress and burnout for individuals and groups. It can also serve to provide peer support and promote change by using the collective voice of the members.
- *Mentor/mentee* systems can facilitate personal and professional development of both parties. An experienced nurse acting as mentor can guide and help a less experienced nurse to gain confidence and skills in her work. This relationship may involve observation, working together and discussion. In this way, both nurses are required to consider how they feel and how they appear to each other, on a regular basis.
- Good *physical* and *mental health* promote self-confidence. It is important to recognise their value, often taken for granted, and to channel energy into maintaining a comfortable balance. Physical exercise can also be an effective

form of tension release, e.g. walking, cycling, jogging, aerobics, dancing, tennis, though excessive exercise can be a symptom of stress.

● Coping with a problem requires *problem-solving* ability. Difficulties often occur with identifying the exact nature of the problem, e.g. what are the problems in this situation? Which problems do I have to deal with? When do I have to deal with them? Who can deal with the others? What are my priorities? If the steps of the problem-solving cycle are followed, this can promote good decisions based upon good assessment of the problem (see, for example, Porritt 1984).

Problem solving is a key indirect coping skill. Bond (1986) devotes an entire chapter to creative problem solving, focusing upon rational and intuitive thinking. Her problem-solving, suggestion is to construct 'thought-maps'. This is a particularly helpful way of linking one's thoughts into a problem-solving pattern. Creative problem solving encourages scope for individual flair, and can be an enjoyable challenge. Having solved a problem once, does the person continue to use the same coping on subsequent occasions? Repetition is not always appropriate, and consideration of alternative strategies permits more flexibility.

Assertiveness

Bond (1986) suggests that 'non-assertive approaches can lead you to further stress, because of lack of respect from other people, not having your needs met and from feeling bad about yourself'. The emphasis includes how a person feels about herself. For example, do you feel that you have a right to state your own needs, to be treated with respect, to express your views, and to make mistakes? Assertiveness involves expression of beliefs in rights without undue emotion or aggression (Porritt 1984). Both body and verbal language express assertiveness.

It is often difficult to say 'no' to a senior colleague, yet the consequences of saying 'yes' should be considered. One strategy for saying 'no' is to be pleasant, clear and honest, for example 'I can see that you need help but I'm busy for the next half-hour.' Explanations and alternatives may or may not be appropriate, e.g. 'I'm in the middle of changing Mr. X's dressing. I could help you afterwards.'

In Lathlean *et al.*'s (1986) study, new nurses identified unfair criticism and lack of feedback as stressful. The ideal here is for the nurse to receive and to give others constructive criticism. Porritt (1984) suggests a strategy for giving feedback including, first, the acknowledgement of the good points, followed by the specific description of the behaviours that appear to need changing, and, finally, the encouragement of the person to think of her own solutions while offering self as a support if necessary. Conversely, the individual should view such criticism of value in contributing to self-awareness, and Porritt (1984) argues that the person should try to hear the feedback without becoming defensive, and in turn evaluate the comments made. Clearly, though, the fruitful giving and acceptance of criticism involves mutual trust, understanding and respect, attributes which are sometimes more likely to pertain between peers rather than between people in a hierarchical relationship.

Bond (1986) says that evaluation involves balancing reason and emotion. She argues that one should try to accept what is valid, and challenge what is not, assertively. For example: 'yes I may take more time to change Mr. X's dressing than other nurses, but I think what I do is thorough'. When receiving destructive criticism, Porritt (1984) suggests that the individual protects him or herself in whatever way he or she can. It seems advisable to use assertiveness in a professional manner. Responding in a dignified way may well emphasise the weakness of the destructive approach, and help to maintain self-respect.

Stress control techniques

A number of stress control techniques have been developed to increase coping and enhance control over stress. Their main principle is the development of control over the involuntary sympathetic nervous system through the influence of the central nervous system and extending the somatic functioning of the body (Schwartz 1978 in Bailey 1985). These techniques are described and clear instructions are given by Bailey (1985). He suggests that health professionals should have access to competent therapists who will teach and supervise the practice of these methods, e.g. clinical psychologists, specialist nurses, occupational therapists and physiotherapists.

People can learn to let body and mind relax together, but one of the difficulties that nurses face is the 'busy' syndrome (Bond 1986). This is when being continually busy is valued. However, the busier a person is the more important it is to take time out. This allows for rationalisation and reorganisation if necessary. Separation of work and non-work can be achieved by having a 'decompression' time. A common strategy is to 'relax in a bath' but one nurse in Lathlean et al.'s (1986) study achieved the mental break between work and non-work by carefully going over the events of the day on her way home from work and then 'letting the thoughts go' as she went through the front door.

Awareness of physical and mental tension is important if the need for relaxation is to be recognised. Common sites of tension are the forehead, temple, jaw, neck and shoulders, lower spine and buttocks. Lying or sitting in a comfortable position, and concentrating upon relaxing each of these areas in turn may help to identify the sites of tension. Each set of muscles can be stretched or squeezed for a few seconds followed by relaxation.

Massage, soft music and deep breathing can enhance relaxation. Controlled breathing is a simple yet vital aid to relaxation. Bailey (1985) explains that 'there is clear evidence that the way we breathe influences how we feel, and how we feel influences how we breathe. Correct breathing is the bridge to stress control, and composed professional alertness.' Bailey suggests that observing your breathing generates a stillness, and describes some useful breathing exercises in his book (Bailey 1985).

Support from the organisation

Hingley and Harris (1986) suggest that support within the organisation can come in many forms, for example peer support groups, a professional mentor, a counselling service, education about stress reduction techniques, training to increase stress awareness, professional support systems, role definition and appraisal. McElroy (1982) offers a list of practical solutions that an organisation can employ either to prevent or to alleviate stress. These are shown in Fig. 6.13.

Fig. 6.13   Ways in which organisation can prevent or alleviate stress (Source: McElroy 1982)

- Equalise demands–resources balance.
- Screening coping ability of candidates applying for high stress jobs.
- Promote staff pride by
    competitive selection;
    a distinctive uniform;
    pay differential for hazardous work;
    flexible work schedule.
- Rotation to less stressful areas.
- Team approach
    period of orientation and training;
    sharing difficult tasks;
    staff meetings;
    encourage informal and formal support systems;
    educational programmes in work time.

Peer support groups can provide a social support system – a collective coping strategy. The group explores the demands made on it, how individuals within the group cope and the influence of various efforts to cope on their professional lives (Gillespie and Gillespie 1986). Such groups can be informal coffee-talks or formal networks such as counselling services for individuals and groups, or a form of stress management training.

Some organisations concentrate both resources and effort into looking after heir staff and providing opportunities for them to discuss problems and resolve tress provoking issues. Unfortunately, there is little evidence of sophisticated provision for nurses in UK health care institutions, though the problems are being recognised more than previously. An example of an American consultation service is shown in Fig. 6.14.

Fig. 6.14   Nursing consultation service at Stanford University Hospital (Source: Bailey 1985)

Goals	Facility
1. Promote and strengthen role performance.	1. Single consultations.
2. Confidential listening.	2. Long-term consultations.
3. Problem-solving proficiency.	3. Individual consultations.
4. Resolution of intra- and inter-professional conflict.	4. Group support options.
5. Promoting and maintaining well-being.	5. Workshops on stress, coping and burnout.

Gillespie and Gillespie (1986) suggest that organisations in which nurses work should have stress management programmes based on the following five principles:

. Programmes should be sensitive to the role that individual differences play in defining what is stressful.

. All programmes should assess the nature and quality of the individual nurse's support system, and should ensure that the nurse has the interpersonal skills to nurture and use others in a supportive manner.

. All programmes should foster flexibility in nurses' coping repertoire. It is essential that a simple formula is *not* prescribed for coping with stress.

. Programmes that elicit individual nurses' appraisal regarding stressors, and their ability to handle them, are likely to be most effective (to include nurses' feelings, thoughts, attitudes, past experiences, knowledge of effects and evaluation of the benefits of various actions).

. Programmes need to include assignments in which there are gradual exposures to stressful events, leading to feedback and self-confidence.

Bailey argues that the provision of wide-ranging facilities for all health service personnel, whether they are struggling under stress or functioning healthily, is a positive step towards individual and organisational well-being.

Conclusion

t is important to recognise the individuality of nurses, each with her own perceptions, needs and abilities. Team work requires a group of individuals with different but complementary skills. The newly qualified nurse has special needs in relation to the new role, as well as needs relating to herself as an individual.

By being more aware of stress in herself, and in others, the new nurse can – with help – begin to tackle some of the issues. The first few months as a trained nurse can be quite daunting. McElroy (1982) offers the following suggestion: 'It is essential that the professional nurse be true to herself, that she have realistic expectations and limitations, and that she consider her own feelings important.'

References

Atkinson, R. L., Atkinson, R. C. and Hilgard, E. R. (1983) *Introduction to Psychology*, 8th edn, London: Harcourt, Brace and Jovanovich Ltd.

Bailey, R. D. (1985) *Coping with Stress in Caring*, Oxford: Blackwell Scientific Publications.

Bamber, M. (1988) 'Slant on stress', *Nursing Times*, Vol. 84, No. 11, pp. 61–3.

Binnie, A. J. (1988) *The Working Lives of Staff Nurses: a Sociological Perspective*. Unpublished MSc Thesis, Warwick University.

Bond, M. (1986) *Stress and Self-Awareness: a Guide for Nurses*, London: Heinemann.

Castledine, G. (1988) 'Clinical nurse specialists', *Nursing Practice*, Vol. 1, pp. 213–14.

Clarke, M. (1984) 'Stress and coping: constructs for nursing', *Journal of Advanced Nursing*, Vol. 9, pp. 3–13.

Clarke, M. (1989) *Stress and Coping in Nursing*, London: Chapman Hall.

Cox, T. (1985) *Stress*, 2nd edn, London: Macmillan.

Eliezer, N. (1981) 'The need for support systems for staff in oncology units', in Tiffany R. (ed.) *Cancer Nursing Update*, London: Baillière Tindall.

Folkman, S., Lazarus, R. S., Dunkett-Schetter, C., DeLougis, A. and Gruen, R. J. (1986) 'Dynamics of a stressful encounter: cognitive appraisal, coping and encounter outcomes', *Journal of Personality and Psychology*, Vol. 50, No. 5, pp. 992–1003.

Freudenberger, H. J. (1974) 'Staff burnout', *Journal of Social Issues*, Vol. 30, pp 159–95.

Gillespie, C. and Gillespie, V. (1986) 'Reading the danger signals', *Nursing Times*, Vol 85, No. 28, pp. 24–7.

Hingley, P. (1984) 'The humane face of nursing', *Nursing Mirror*, Vol. 159, No. 21, pp 19–22.

Hingley, P. and Harris, P. (1986) 'Lowering the tension', *Nursing Times*, Vol. 85, No 30, pp. 52–3.

Humphries, A. (1987) *The Transition from Student to Staff Nurse*. Unpublished BSc Thesis, Leicester University.

Lathlean, J., Smith, G. and Bradley, S. (1986) *Post-Registration Development Schemes Evaluation*, Kings College, University of London.

McElroy, A. M. (1982) 'Burnout – a review of the literature with application to cancer nursing', *Cancer Nursing*, June, pp. 211–17.

Newlin, N. J. and Wellisch, D. K. (1978) 'The oncology nurse: life on a roller coaster', *Cancer Nursing*, December, pp. 447–9.

Nichols, K. A., Springford, V. and Searle, J. (1981) 'An investigation of distress and discontent in various types of nursing, *Journal of Advanced Nursing*, Vol. 6, pp. 311–18.

Porritt, L. (1984) *Communication Choices for Nurses*, London: Churchill Livingstone.

Vaughan, B. (1980) *The Newly Qualified Staff Nurse – Factors Affecting Transition*, Unpublished MSc Thesis, University of Manchester.

7 Coping with Death and Dying

JESSICA CORNER

Introduction

Today at least 60 per cent of deaths occur in hospital rather than at home, or in a specialist unit such as a hospice (Parkes 1978). In urban areas it is even higher at around 75 per cent (Taylor 1983). This means that two-thirds of people die in institutions, and a relatively small number of the dying receive specialist terminal care in hospices or under the care of support teams. Dealing with dying patients' physical and psychological needs rests to a great extent with health carers who in the main have had no special training for their role in dying. This can be a frightening and difficult experience for many nurses, doctors, and other health carers, who are left to learn to deal with dying patients with little support.

As Carr (1982, p.217) states: 'This underlines an important feature of dying and death at the present time: they have become unfamiliar events that take place in unfamiliar surroundings, watched over by unfamiliar people.'

Fulton (1976) points out that in the United States the present generation of youth is the first to be 'death free', statistically speaking, in the history of the world. That is, the period of time that a nuclear family can expect not to have death within its ranks due to increasing longevity and better health generally, is now one generation or approximately twenty years. Quint (1967) notes that while young people are exposed to death presented in detail on television and films, they have little opportunity to participate directly in the mourning process and family rituals which were relatively common before the Second World War.

For western societies today, death has become a taboo subject, and the fact that death is the inevitable consequence of living is denied. Euphemisms for dying are used (passed on, gone to rest, etc.); those who are dying are hidden away in institutions, while those who have died are quickly removed. On hospital wards the patients are protected from the knowledge that someone has died, curtains are drawn around beds while the body is removed, and the empty bed quickly re-made and filled with another patient. This only serves to prevent patients expressing their anxiety and sadness when a fellow patient dies.

150

Fulton (1976) outlines some of the reasons for such denial of death. With advances in medical science premature death has become a relatively rare phenomenon, death being confined to the elderly. Death has also become institutionalised into hospitals. This is in sharp contrast to Victorian society where life expectancy was shorter, many families experienced the death of children and young adults, and death occurred at home with family around. There were also many ritualised practices surrounding death, with elaborate funeral processions and long periods of mourning for close relatives. As society has become more secularised and religion plays a much smaller part in our lives, death has increasingly been pushed aside. Society's emphasis on youth and beauty allows no place for death.

A rotten way to die?'

The article 'A rotten way to die' appeared in the *Guardian's* 'Society Tomorrow' page in September 1986 (see Fig. 7.1). In it Alison Wertheimer describes her mother's last few days of life which she spent on a busy hospital ward before being transferred to a hospice for her final twenty-four hours. The contrast between care on the hospital ward and in the hospice is striking, and yet the scene is alarmingly familiar and could have happened on almost any ward in any hospital. Alison Wertheimer ends by calling for the principles of hospice care to become part of hospital care for the dying, a question that will be explored later in this chapter.

The 'rotten way to die' described by Alison Wertheimer is one where death appeared to be seen as failure rather than a logical conclusion to a full life, where pain and symptom control were prevented by fears of addiction to drugs, and the needs of both patient and family were neglected among the more pressing concerns of a busy National Health Service ward.

There is, however, another side to the story. It is not only Alison Wertheimer and her mother who have felt caught in a system designed to 'deal' with death. Many nurses also find caring for dying patients difficult, and that preparation for this important role during training is inadequate.

Nurses' feelings about the care of dying patients

In the 1960s Jeane Quint (1967) undertook a sociological study in which she looked at the social phenomenon of dying. She focused on how student nurses learn about dying patients in five schools of nursing around San Francisco. Quint found that there was little emphasis on teaching student nurses to care for, or planning for students to be assigned to, dying patients during their training. Some students qualified without witnessing death or participating in terminal care. The emphasis was on life saving procedures and on 'cure'. The

Fig. 7.1 'A rotten way to die' (Source: Wertheimer 1986)

'When we finally arrived, we were taken to a gloomy single room. The bedside bell was broken. As my mother's cancer meant she could by then only whisper, she would have been helpless if left alone.' Alison Wertheimer wonders why it was necessary for her mother to escape from hospital to be granted a dignified death.'

A rotten way to die

Eighteen months ago my mother was dying of cancer in a large London teaching hospital, waiting for a bed at the nearest hospice. A bed was available just in time. She died less than 24 hours after arriving there and I still breathe a sigh of relief that she didn't die in that hospital. Perhaps we were just unlucky with that particular hospital (although, ironically, my mother had chosen to work there as a nurse for five years). But I am still left wondering how they managed to get so much wrong – and the hospice managed to get it right. I'm still wondering if it's really only hospices that can provide good terminal care and if hospitals can't learn some of the lessons that hospices have to offer.

When you're going somewhere to die, how you're treated on arrival seems important. Leaving home for the last time wasn't easy for my mother, in spite of the kindness of the ambulancemen. Our arrival at the hospital did nothing to lessen our collective depression though. Although the admission had been arranged earlier that day, the bed wasn't ready and we weren't allowed up to the ward. Instead we spent a miserable half-hour stuck in a corner of the very busy casualty department. Doctors and nurses rushed around but no one took any notice of us – until I insisted on being taken up to the ward.

When we finally arrived, we were taken to a gloomy single room. It wasn't very clean; but worse still, the bedside call bell was broken. As my mother's cancer meant she could by then only whisper, she would have been helpless if left alone.

For the next few hours nurses dashed briefly in and out, never stopping to talk for long but throwing out cheery remarks like 'Oh good; now you're back we can feed you up a bit.' Maybe they hadn't read her notes and maybe they didn't notice she was dying but the feeble jokes and lack of awareness of her situation made her, and me, very angry. It took five hours for a doctor to arrive so during that time no medication was allowed. He was young and rather nervous. He didn't want to prescribe anything much 'in case she got used to it'. (I suppose they could have written 'drug addiction' instead of 'cancer' on the death certificate. Would it have mattered?)

Over the next two days my mother, who had been calm and peaceful before we arrived at the hospital, became increasingly angry and depressed. Misery was compounded by a sense of isolation, and it seemed as though the staff were unable or unwilling to share in what we were going through. On a busy hospital ward maybe the staff don't have too much time to talk, but it was hard not to feel that we were getting little attention because there wasn't much they felt they could offer a dying person. At one point I did suggest tentatively to one of the doctors that it would be better for everyone when we could move to the hospice. Her response that 'we do deal with it here, you know', didn't leave me feeling any more optimistic about their ability to do more than deal with death.

Perhaps it is hard for hospitals when they can't actively 'treat' people any more; but there were so many small things they could have done which would have made a world of difference. The offering of food, for example, has always been one of the best ways we can show care for another person. My mother didn't want, or need, very much to eat by then, but when a full portion of not very attractively served food was just slapped down on a table – often out of her reach – she usually ended up not touching most of the meal; not that anyone seemed to mind, despite the talk about 'feeding her up'.

Being a visitor in hospital is, at the best times, a strange

Fig. 7.1 (contd)

experience, but sitting by the hospital bed I began to wonder if I was invisible. I used to arrive on the ward at breakfast-time. Sometimes a nurse would say hello, but otherwise nobody really seemed to acknowledge my presence. I wasn't even sure I was supposed to be there outside the official visiting hours. No one questioned me so I stayed, but a positive welcome would have been nice. Although I was sometimes there for seven or eight hours, no one suggested I might like to use the hospital dining facilities which must have existed. I suppose I could have eaten my mother's untouched meals though I'm sure that would have been against the rules; it felt demeaning having to beg a cup of tea or coffee from the trolley lady.

Two days before my mother died I came on the ward to find her utterly defeated. Convinced she wouldn't make it to the hospice where a bed was free the following day, and barely able to hold a pen she wrote a note, insisting I give it to one of the nurses. She begged them to 'let her go,' saying 'I can't stand it any longer.' I'm pretty sure that it wasn't physical pain that was troubling her but I couldn't explain to the staff that it was being in hospital that had brought her to write that note.

It was a young student nurse who dealt with my tears, calmed my mother down and told me that she'd give up nursing the day she stopped caring about her patients. It was the first time I felt anyone in that huge institution really cared about what we were going through.

Our arrival at the hospice the next day was a complete contrast to the hospital. Matron was waiting with the welcome 'I'm so glad you've chosen to come and be with us'; and her bed was waiting by the front door, warmed with a homely hot-water bottle.

On the ward, over morning coffee served to both of us, staff came in and introduced themselves and helped us settle in. I say 'us' because that's how it was in the hospice; there wasn't just a 'patient', but rather a dying person and their family who were all involved.

The doctor arrived within half an hour, not really for a consultation but more of a chat. It was so unlike the one brief visit we'd had from a consultant in hospital who had come in, and without introducing herself roughly examined my mother and disappeared. This doctor managed to examine her with minimum disturbance but more importantly, we were communicating for the first time with openness about what was happening. No miracles were offered, mind you, but my mother was gently promised 'you will not die in distress and you will not die alone.' It was worth a thousand 'treatments' to see her calmness returning.

At the hospice relatives are given a great deal of care and attention. There was, for example, no question of my sitting hungry by the bedside. While my mother was given a small and dainty lunch (almost the first meal she'd eaten for several days), I was taken down to the dining room to lunch with the nurses. My offer of payment for the meal was gently but firmly refused. Hospice hospitality is important and they believe in looking after families too. We had endless time and attention from the staff generally, both during that day and after my mother died.

Much of what we experienced at that hospice could I'm sure be replicated in hospital settings. That seems to be important, because although the hospice movement is growing fast, the fact remains that in the foreseeable future more people will die in hospital than in hospices. Hospices have already been able to teach the hospitals a great deal about such matters as pain relief and control. But if hospitals are going to do more than just 'deal with death' they still have a lot of learning to do.

nurses worked in ward environments where non-involvement with patients self-control and 'coping' with any situation were characteristics that were highly valued. Students often learnt to model their behaviour on more senior nurses who avoided relatives and potentially disturbing conversations with dying patients.

Some of the most extreme and shocking experiences nurses had were during their encounters with death. These could be turning points in their lives, leaving the student with an overwhelming sense of success or failure. The student's first encounter with death seemed to be particularly significant and lasting impressions were held of the event. These impressions were influenced by the expectedness of the death, the perceived suffering of the patient and the support the students had from other staff at the time. Quint also found that concerns relating to caring for the dying changed in the newly qualified staff nurse as they were faced for the first time with deciding how to cope with difficult families or decisions over whether to resuscitate when they felt the patient ought to be allowed to die in peace.

Birch (1983) assessed 207 student and pupil nurses' levels of anxiety in their first and second years of hospital experience, from four schools of nursing in the north of England. The nurses answered questionnaires which asked them to rate how anxious they felt about fifty-six areas of clinical practice from basic tasks, for example disposal of urine, to aspects of death and dying, abortion and relief of pain. Birch repeated the assessment, at eight-monthly intervals, for two years. There were a number of areas which the nurses rated as consistently stressful as the student and pupil nurses progressed through their training. It is interesting to note that six out of thirteen of these highly stressful areas related to dealing with aspects of dying and bereavement. Birch concluded that behavioural aspects of care, particularly those which related to death and dying are a major source of anxiety to learner nurses.

In Lathlean et al.'s (1986) study of newly registered staff nurses over 80 per cent of the ninety-two staff nurses who completed questionnaires at the end of their first six months as staff nurses, felt they needed to learn at least some aspects of dealing with dying patients and their relatives, and 45 per cent felt they needed to learn a great deal. Over 50 per cent felt that it was a stressful and problematic area of their role. There is now a body of evidence which suggests that the care dying patients receive is less than adequate, and that the needs of the dying and their relatives both before and after death are not being met.

Drummond-Mills (1983) observed patients in their last week of life in four large teaching hospitals in Glasgow and looked at nurses and medical staff interacting with patients. She revealed that:

- Overall the care for the dying was inadequate.
- The nursing services were governed by routine and the care was given predominantly by junior nurses.

- Patients were often left alone, and only had brief contact with nurses no more than once or twice an hour, and had minimal contact with doctors.
- Patients who were admitted to die received fewer visits and less nursing time than patients admitted with a more positive diagnosis.
- 65 per cent of the patients were conscious and aware that they were dying.

Knight and Field (1981) observed the communication patterns of nurses with terminal cancer patients on an acute surgical ward. The ward held a general policy of not informing the patient he/she was dying. This meant that patients had to rely heavily on their ability to recognise their physical deterioration if they were to become aware of their impending death. Once patients with inoperable cancer returned to the ward from the theatre and their drugs had been prescribed, the doctors rarely asked them more than 'Are you in pain?' The question of going home was avoided, as was any discussion with the patient about the operation. The care of the dying fell largely by default to first year student nurses. These junior nurses had greatest contact with dying patients and, by the nature of their work, formed deep and difficult relationships with them. These nurses commonly used two strategies to avoid answering patient's questions. First, the ward organisation made it possible for them to be doing work elsewhere and thus to avoid contact with patients, or to suggest by their actions that they were too busy to talk. Second, they would use their low status in the ward hierarchy to plead ignorance of the patient's case and refer the patient on to more senior staff (usually the doctor) who were then never called.

Quint (1965) observed communication patterns of nurses and doctors with women undergoing mastectomy, and found that cultural attitudes towards cancer and death were reflected in doctors' and nurses' behaviour. These women were not well informed about their cancer and the surgical procedure. What they were told was couched in generalities rather than telling them about the relative success of the surgery or the extent of cancer involvement found. Physicians and nurses made it difficult for the women to ask questions. These barriers to verbal communication were noticeably higher the more extensive the cancer involvement. The word 'cancer' was avoided at all times. Nurses avoided these patients by using gestures and actions that made it difficult for a patient to initiate conversation (like looking very busy), and they interrupted the patient in conversation if talk threatened to get out of hand by focusing directly on either diagnosis or prognosis. Patient contact was primarily to perform tasks except where the patient was obviously liked by staff. It was evident that preferred patients were those who handled their illness in a way which was not disturbing to staff. The nurses used tactics which directed discussion with these patients into safe areas by focusing on the procedure the nurse was doing (for example a dressing, or intravenous infusion) or small talk (e.g. chatting about the weather). They were seldom encouraged to talk about their illness or cancer.

Sometimes a patient asked a direct question, for example 'Am I going to die?' Here nurses reported using tactics to avoid giving a direct answer, by changing the subject, lapsing into silence or making such inappropriate statements as 'We all have to go sometime'. Nurses also did not routinely ask physicians for specific information about the possibility of metastases. This protected them from feelings of sadness and it also made it easier to respond to patients' questions with 'I don't know'. Quint concluded that while the central issue that these women faced was the possibility of death, most faced it alone because family and friends as well as doctors and nurses blocked them from discussing it.

Webster (1981) found that many student nurses described stressful situations they had encountered while caring for the dying. Over 30 per cent of the nurses in her study claimed that they were not always even told which patients were expected to die, and they were even less likely to be told whether or not the patient had been told he was dying. Education for students on caring for the dying was not a routine part of the curriculum but depended on individual tutors, many of whom in the study did not include it in what they taught students. It was anticipated that students would pick up the necessary skills by working alongside more experienced staff nurses. Yet when Margaret Webster observed practices on the ward 25 per cent of the learners worked unaccompanied with dying patients. Both the learners and the trained nurses she observed seemed to have difficulties in communicating with dying patients, and in only four cases did she observe that patients were encouraged to talk about their illness, ask questions or express feelings.

The physical needs of dying patients

It is not only communicating and the psychological care of dying patients that are problematic. There is also evidence that nurses are not meeting the physical needs of dying patients either.

Twycross and Lack (1983) estimate that a minimum of 25 per cent of all cancer patients die without relief from severe pain. Parkes (1978) interviewed spouses whose partners had died of cancer in two South London Boroughs between 1967 and 1971. Of the patients who had died in hospital, 46 per cent of their spouses were critical of the care they had received. Twenty per cent were said to have suffered severe and mostly continuous pain and several patients had been greatly distressed by unrelieved dyspnoea. Other complaints related to lack of support and contact with medical and nursing staff.

Jennifer Hunt's (1977) study of patients with protracted pain at the London Hospital gives us some insight into the reasons for inadequate pain relief. She considered that:

● Patients' expectations were too low, they praised doctors and nurses despite in many cases still being in pain.

- A high proportion of patients were on 'as required' prescriptions.
- Of those patients receiving analgesics regularly, a number were still in pain indicating that doctors fail to appreciate that effective analgesia varies from patient to patient.
- Nurses accepted the presence of unrelieved pain too readily. They did not assess pain between drug rounds and failed to pick up cues indicating that the patients may still be in pain.
- Nurses failed to recognise the importance of their own contribution to relief of pain.
- More education on pain relief was urgently needed for both doctors and nurses.

There is some evidence to suggest that the gap between hospice care for the dying and that provided by general hospitals is narrowing (Parkes 1984). There have been attempts to reproduce the hospice model of care in general hospitals in the form of symptom control teams and continuing care units based within the National Health Service. There has also been a move towards caring for the dying at home with the support of hospital and hospice-based home care teams and day care in continuing care units and hospices. It is both cheaper and, for many patients, more comfortable to be in their own homes with their family and personal possessions around them. This is not possible, though, for all patients, particularly the elderly and those living alone. Home care for the dying also places considerable strain on relatives, and good symptom control has in the past been more difficult to achieve at home. Since the majority of dying patients will continue to be cared for in general hospitals it is essential that nurses gain confidence and skills in caring for the dying.

Fig. 7.2 gives a summary of the difficulties expressed by groups of newly registered nurses in caring for dying patients.

This chapter aims to provide information for you to help deal with these areas of difficulty. Resource lists of further reading and agencies are provided where further information and help can be found.

Returning to Alison Wertheimer's call for the principles of hospice care to become part of hospital care for the dying, the hospice principle involves the following:

good symptom control;
- a supportive, open and informal atmosphere;
- maximum participation of relatives in care and the ward/hospice environment;
continuity of care.

The concept of continuing care is also important. This means that the above principles should be applied from the outset when the patient first receives a

Fig. 7.2   Nurses' difficulties in dealing with dying patients

Nurses expressed feelings of 'inadequacy' to deal with:
- The patient's and family's emotional needs.
- Control of the patient's pain and other symptoms.
- Ethical issues such as:
    to tell or not to tell the patient they are dying;
    what to do if relatives or the consultant does not want the
    patient told;
    how to answer difficult questions from patients.
- Bereavement and anticipatory grief in relatives.

They also highlighted their own:
- Lack of knowledge
- Lack of counselling skills

in relation to the dying process and how to communicate with dying patients.

diagnosis of a terminal illness, through to the patient's eventual death maintaining the highest quality of life, preferably at home with intermittent admissions to hospital during exacerbation of symptoms, and/or to provide respite care for relatives.

This may all seem impossible to achieve if the ward sister or consultant does not agree with telling patients/or talking to patients about dying; the ward is drastically understaffed, or if it is felt that neither the nurses nor the doctor have enough knowledge of pain and symptom control. The first step, though, is to feel confident in one's own personal knowledge and ability to deal with the patient's physical and psychological problems. Staff nurses *are* in a position to influence prescriptions of drugs for patients and also act as a role model for more junior nurses, with the potential to be highly influential in relation to the quality of care on their ward.

Many nurses feel that their training, with its emphasis on physical aspects of care, has adequately equipped them for their role in caring for the dying. This may be so, but when questioned more closely they would not know what specifically to suggest a junior doctor do if for instance a dying patient was in pain, or how best to deal with a dying lung cancer patient's dyspnoea. This chapter cannot provide all the answers, but some basic principles of control for common symptoms of dying patients are discussed. There are many very good texts on the subject available to provide a comprehensive picture of pain and symptom control.

Pain control

The increased understanding of the principles of pain control which has come about as a result of the hospice movement largely relates to pain in cancer patients. This is because pain is a common symptom in cancer patients with advanced disease. Figures showing the symptoms of patients admitted to Sir Michael Sobell House, a hospice in Oxford, show that 60–70 per cent of patients admitted have pain. This figure is likely to overestimate pain in cancer patients though since one of the functions of the hospice is to deal with difficult pain problems (Hanks 1983).

This discussion on pain control is derived from research into cancer patients, but what is really being talked about is the difference between acute and chronic pain. It is the cause of the specific pain which dictates the appropriate treatment and not the fact that it is a cancer pain, a heart pain or an arthritis pain.

Hanks (1983) has summarised the differences between acute and chronic pain. This is illustrated in Fig. 7.3. This means that the chronic pain seen in dying patients is likely to present in different ways from a patient in acute pain, for instance after surgery, or the pain of childbirth or toothache. The patient in chronic pain is not likely to be writhing in agony clutching the painful limb or muscle, but may appear depressed, withdrawn and describe symptoms of sleeplessness or anorexia. The symptoms of chronic pain resemble depression. As demonstrated by Hanks (1985) pain is not just the perception of a painful stimulus but is also the emotional reaction to that perception. The pain of the dying patient is likely to elicit negative emotions depending on its meaning to the individual. This emotional component to the dying patient's pain can be very apparent and pain is therefore likely to vary.

Fig. 7.3   Differences between acute and chronic pain (After Hanks 1983)

Acute pain	Chronic pain
Event	Situation
Duration predictable and limited	Duration unpredictable
Tends to get better	Tends to get worse
Has meaning and purpose	Has no meaning or a negative meaning

A second and important point in dealing with dying patient's pain is the importance of adequate assessment. There is a tendency to use the following formula:

DYING PATIENT + PAIN = OPIATE ANALGESIC
= 10 mg MORPHINE EVERY 4 HOURS

This blanket approach to pain is wrong. In a study of 100 cancer patients in pain admitted to the Oxford Hospice, Sir Michael Sobell House (Twycross and Lack

1983), it was found that the number of anatomically distinct pains in each patient ranged from one to eight; eighty of the patients had more than one distinct pain and thirty-four had four or more. Another important finding was that in less than half of the patients the cancer alone caused the pain. Constipation, pressure sores, arthritis and even ordinary headaches contributed in these patients' pain. This is important since pain caused by different processes requires different treatments, and arthritis and headaches are certainly not best treated by morphine or diamorphine.

Pain may also change during the dying process; different pains may emerge and others disappear. This highlights the need for continuous assessment and review of pain.

The use of a pain assessment chart like that in Fig. 7.4 may be helpful. This allows the patient to indicate on the body outlines each distinct pain, and also the pain scale enables the patient to indicate both its nature and intensity. Analgesics prescribed can be recorded and their effects on each pain site (labelled a–h) noted. A section for social and emotional factors, patient activity and pain, and things the patient has found of benefit is included.

There are a number of points to bear in mind when caring for patients in pain which relate to the prescription of analgesics. While nurses would not normally see prescription as part of their role, an understanding of the principles of pain control used in conjunction with an assessment tool can be helpful when liaising with the medical team.

It is important to give analgesics, including the opiods like morphine, as early as necessary in the course of the patient's disease. There has often been a reluctance to do this with patients due to fears of addiction, respiratory depression, accepting what the patients says hurts, and fears about what to give the patient at the end if he is started on opiates too early. All of these fears are unfounded as will be seen later.

Patients who are dying and in pain do not automatically need strong opiods like morphine and diamorphine. They do if they have severe pain. For mild pain a non-opiod such as aspirin or paracetamol may be enough, but most patients with mild to moderate pain will require a weak opiod such as codeine or coproxamol. If a patient is in pain whilst taking a weak opiod regularly there is little point in changing to another weak opiod, for instance dihydrocodeine to coproxamol, since the potency of the two drugs is similar. This will not achieve pain control. If the patient's pain is not relieved it is logical to move the patient on to a strong opiod such as morphine. This helps to keep drug therapy simple and effective. On the whole, elaborate concoctions of different weak opiods are unlikely to help, and side-effects and drug interactions are more likely.

There has in the past been a reluctance to prescribe strong opiods because of fears of the following:

- respiratory depression;
- addiction;
- tolerance.

Fig. 7.4   (a) p.1 of the revised pain chart; (b) p.2 of the revised pain chart; (c) p.3 of the revised pain chart (Source: Walker and Dicks 1987)

PAIN ASSESSMENT CHART

SURNAME: HOSPITAL NO.

FIRST NAME: DATE:

INITIAL ASSESSMENT

Patient's own description of the pain(s):

What helps relieve the pain?

What makes the pain worse?

Do you have pain

i)   at night?   Yes/No (comment if required).

ii)   at rest?   Yes/No (comment if required)

iii)   on movement?   Yes/No (comment if required)

(a)

PAIN SITES

Please draw on the body outlines below to show where you feel pain.   Label each site of pain with a letter A, B, C, etc.

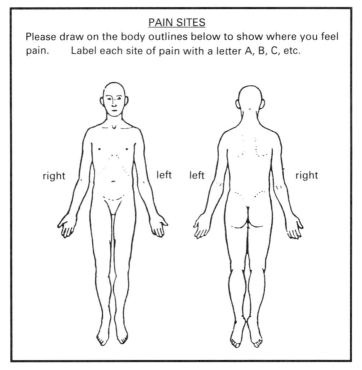

(b)

PAIN ASSESSMENT CHART

KEY TO PAIN INTENSITY

0 = no pain   4 = very severe pain
1 = mild pain   5 = intolerable/overwhelming pain
2 = moderate pain
3 = severe pain   s = sleeping

it may be easier to determine the intensity of pain by looking at the pain scale below.

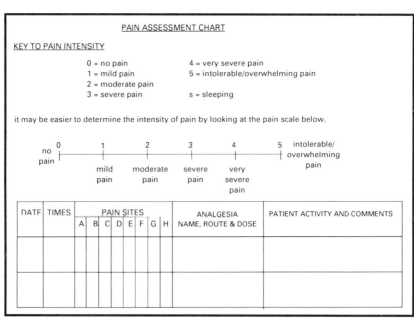

(c)

These fears are largely unfounded. *Respiratory depression* is not a problem because 'pain is the physiological antagonist of the depressant effects of opiod analgesics' (Hanks 1983).

This means that pain cancels out the depressant effects of such drugs as morphine. In this way if the dose of morphine is gradually increased upwards until the point at which the patient is no longer in pain, respiratory depression will not occur. Only if the patient is given too high a dose, or if for some reason the pain disappears (perhaps through some other treatment such as surgery, a nerve block, or radiotherapy) will respiratory depression occur.

Addiction is also not a problem, since the psychological dependance or 'drug craving' seen in dying addicts does not occur. Physical dependence does occur, but again it is not the problem seen in drug addicts and many patients have successfully weaned themselves off morphine without any problem when they found they did not need it any longer. *Tolerance* does sometimes occur, but it is simply dealt with by increasing the dose of morphine. Morphine also does not precipitate the patient's death. Administration of morphine is *not euthanasia*; if given appropriately a patient who dies soon after being started on morphine would have died anyway. The drug does not hasten the end.

The concept of prophylactic analgesia

It is cruel to wait for pain to return or for the next drug round before giving the next dose of analgesia. In order to control pain effectively it is important to eradicate the patient's memory of the pain. It is most unpleasant for patients to have pain relieved knowing that it will be back in a few hours' time. It is also likely that higher doses of analgesics will be required to relieve pain that is allowed to return before subsequent doses of analgesics are given and more side-effects occur.

The time between doses of analgesics depends on the plasma half-life of the drug being used (or the time elapsing before concentration of the drug in plasma is reduced by half its original quantity). For morphine it is three to five hours, so a four-hourly drug regime is appropriate. Fig. 7.5 shows how an 'as required' regular medication allows the concentration of the drug in the plasma to fall below the level required for pain relief. This is compared to a four-hourly drug regime for morphine sulphate. Morphine does have side-effects of constipation, drowsiness, nausea and vomiting. Possible methods of dealing with these are shown in Fig. 7.6.

What should be the dose?

As discussed earlier the starting dose should represent an increment on what the patient has been taking; 10 mg every four hours is the usual starting dose for

Fig. 7.5   The time between analgesic doses (Source: Twycross and Lack 1983)

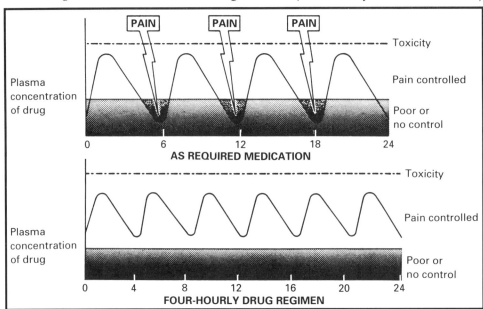

Fig. 7.6   Side effects of morphine and diamorphine

Constipation	Should be treated prophylactically since morphine slows gut motility. Problems usually occur in patients who have not been given an aperient from day one.
Drowsiness	Does occur, but disappears after 2–3 days unless the dose is too high. Patients should be warned of this.
Nausea and vomiting	Occurs in about two-thirds of patients. Haloeperidol 1.5 mg nocte or metoclopramide 20 mg 6 hourly can be useful for this.

patients who have been on a weak opiod. There is no upper limit to the amount of morphine/diamorphine that can be given, so the dose can be adjusted gradually upwards until the patient's pain is controlled.

It is a good idea to break objectives of pain control into stages for the patient, e.g. (Hanks 1985):

PAIN FREE AT NIGHT
PAIN FREE AT REST
PAIN FREE ON MOVEMENT

It is almost always possible to achieve the first two, but for a few patients freedom from pain on movement may be more difficult to achieve.

It is usual to have a second 'breakthrough' dose of morphine written up on the 'as required' section of the patient's drug chart. This should be the same dose as the patient is having regularly. This can be safely given if the patient's pain returns between four-hourly doses. When controlling the patient's pain the number of breakthrough doses required in twenty-four hours can be added to give the amount required every four hours, and this gives an estimate of the patient's requirements. The regular doses of morphine should still be given even though the patient has had a breakthrough dose.

Route of administration

Oral medication is preferable and is suitable for the majority of patients. This prevents trauma from injection and helps the patient maintain his own independence. Other routes may have to be found, for instance in patients with obstruction. But the rectal route, or a syringe driver connected to a subcutaneous injection site should be considered rather than four-hourly injections.

Consider co-analgesics

'A co-analgesic is any drug (or device) which may not have an intrinsic analgesic activity but which when used with a conventional analgesic will contribute significantly to pain relief' (Hanks 1983). Other measures which may significantly improve pain include the following:

- radiotherapy;
- chemotherapy;
- palliative surgery;
- nerve blocks;
- transcutaneous nerve stimulation (battery-operated electrical nerve stimulation);
- massage;
- heat/cold;
- relaxation/hypnotherapy;
- acupuncture;
- discussion of fears/anxieties;
- diversional measures, e.g. art, music, poetry, talking;
- psychological support.

The list is endless and it is here that the nurse's role is very important since many of these measures, such as diversion, relaxation, massage and psychological support, can be employed by nurses in the relief of pain. Nurses need to become much more expert in the use of such techniques. Margo McCaffery's book *Nursing the Patient in Pain* (1979) gives an excellent discussion of the nurse's role in pain control.

Other physical symptoms

Other common symptoms of the dying include the following:

- anorexia;
- constipation;
- dry mouth;
- nausea;
- vomiting;
- dyspnoea;
- oedema;
- insomnia;
- weakness.

There is much that can be done for these symptoms, both as nursing interventions and with pharmacological measures. Assessment of causative and contributory factors is essential. A good example of this is in the use of anti-emetics for the treatment of nausea and vomiting in the dying, since the cause of the problem will determine the appropriate anti-emetic drug.

Nausea and vomiting are initiated centrally via the chemoreceptor trigger zone (CTZ) in the medulla and the vomiting centre in the midbrain; this is stimulated via the CTZ. Anti-emetics tend to act predominantly either on the vomiting centre or the CTZ. For this reason an understanding of how causes of nausea and vomiting act centrally on the CTZ and vomiting centre will determine which drug is most appropriate (Hanks 1983).

Toxic substances in the bloodstream and radiation (e.g. metabolites of drugs and in ureamia, hypercalcaemia) stimulate the CTZ which acts via the vomiting centre to cause nausea and vomiting. But unpleasant sights and smells affecting the higher centres of the brain, or stimuli from the pharynx, heart or gut via the vagus nerve directly affect the vomiting centre.

Haloperidol and Metoclopramide are therefore more appropriate for nausea associated with morphine and ureamia, and cyclizine for intestinal obstruction or raised intracranial pressure. Nursing assessment of the cause of nausea and vomiting, followed by referral to the medical team for appropriate prescription, then careful nursing implementation to help with diet and comfort can do much to alleviate this.

Anorexia and oral symptoms such as dry mouth may also be looked at in a similar way. Careful assessment will reveal whether any of the following are important. Fig. 7.7 illustrates the multitude of different factors which may alone or in combination cause a symptom such as anorexia and intervention for each.

Fig. 7.7   Causes of anorexia and some appropriate interventions (After Twycross and Lack 1984)

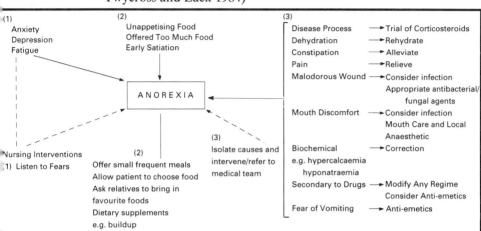

The same kind of approach can be used when assessing patients and deciding on the nursing that is needed, for example with dyspnoea, sleep and oral problems. (Further reading on symptom control is given at the end of this chapter.)

Dealing with the patient's psychological needs

As has been shown by the research into the needs of newly qualified nurses, this is an area which nurses find particularly difficult and worrying. Training in the past has tended to emphasise physical rather than emotional care and it is in the area of dealing with dying patients and grieving relatives that newly registered nurses feel particularly vulnerable. For the first time they may be dealing with death and bereavement without more experienced people around to offer advice and help. There are many good books and articles written on the subject and again the reader is referred to them for a more comprehensive picture (see Further Reading).

The dying process

Much research has been done into coping with a terminal illness and the process of dying. Interest has mushroomed since Glaser and Strauss (1965 and 1968) reported their early work into the process of dying. This was closely followed by Kubler Ross' authoritative work *On Death and Dying* in 1969.

Glaser and Strauss (1965) observed behaviour between hospital staff and dying patients, and the degree of openness that existed about the patient's anticipated death. They documented different levels of awareness. Closed awareness occurred where the patient was kept totally unaware of his prognosis. This was only possible where the patient was not able to recognise his own physical deterioration and where relatives and staff prevented him from 'finding out'. More common was suspected awareness, where the patient was suspicious of his condition, and mutual pretence awareness where both patient and staff were aware that the patient was dying but did not show it to each other. This could be extremely difficult to maintain and caused considerable strain to patients, relatives and staff. Open awareness occurred where patient and staff were aware and were able to communicate openly about it with each other. This level of awareness, while preferable, was not without its problems.

Glaser and Strauss (1968) documented trajectories of dying, that is the physical decline in patients that may be defined as the dying process. Different patterns of decline can represent different difficulties for patients, families and staff coping with dying. On diagnosis of a terminal illness the predicted prognosis (which may or may not be communicated to the patient) allows an estimate of the rate of anticipated physical decline. The concept of dying trajectory is useful since Glaser and Strauss noted that adjustment in patients, relatives and staff only appeared to be facilitated where the patient adhered to the dying trajectory. Many patients, however, do not and this can cause problems. The patient may decline more rapidly than expected, making it difficult for relatives and staff to adjust and preparations to be undertaken. If the patient lingers beyond the time expected this can place considerable strain on families. Occasionally, a seriously ill patient can commence a rapid decline, and then suddenly improve for some length of time before declining again (Lazarus Syndrome). This can cause difficulties when patient and family have prepared for death, made financial arrangements and withdrawn from relationships only to find the patient recovers sufficiently to start 'life' again.

There has been considerable debate over how much openness there should be with terminally ill patients about their impending death. Kubler Ross's (1969) interviews with 400 dying patients revealed that the vast majority of patients actually knew that they were dying regardless of whether they had been formally told or not. They picked up the information through the actions of relatives, doctors and other hospital staff towards them, and from their own physical signs and symptoms. Kubler Ross felt that by allowing patients to talk and being a sensitive listener they will establish for themselves what is true. Most patients will know at some level that they are dying. For this reason an open and supportive atmosphere where patients can express their own thoughts, fears and emotions seems most appropriate.

A number of authors have looked at the process of adaptation to awareness of dying which occurs in patients. This bears a close resemblance to the process of adapting to losses of all kinds be it through bereavement, change in body image, redundancy or dying, and has tended to be described in terms of sequential stages through which individuals pass before adaptation to the loss occurs. Lindeman (1944), Bowlby (1961), Kubler Ross (1969) and Parkes (1972) are some examples. It is important to note, however, that there is little research evidence to suggest that these emotional responses to the process of adaptation to loss and dying actually occur in predictable sequence or stages. The processes described by authors such as Kubler Ross are useful in understanding patients' emotional responses however.

Kubler Ross identified the following stages:

- Denial (as if the patient is saying, 'No, not me')
- Anger ('Why me?')
- Bargaining ('Yes me but . . .')
- Depression ('Yes me'); and
- Acceptance ('It's O.K.')

Table 7.1 outlines how these emotional responses may be manifested in the dying and some possible interventions for dealing with them.

It is difficult to define patients' emotional responses as any particular 'stage' and patients do not necessarily progress through the stages in a logical sequence – they may progress and regress, or fixate at one stage. They may well fluctuate through a variety of coping mechanisms.

Aspects of anger, denial, bargaining, depression and acceptance or resignation may be seen at once. All the emotional responses described by authors such as Kubler Ross represent healthy coping mechanisms and there is really nothing to say that one stage is necessarily better than another. Denial is a healthy coping mechanism too. The idea that a patient has 'accepted' his or her death is not particularly helpful since it assumes that, firstly, acceptance is somehow a better state for the patient to be in, and, secondly, that the patient has finished the process of adaptation. This is often not the case. Few people can face the inevitability of death all of the time; it is too enormous. It also assumes that a 'good' death, whatever that means, can only be achieved if the patient has accepted his death. Some patients never 'accept', while others may simply become resigned to their fate and feel tired with the struggle for life.

Fears of the dying

The dying patient faces many fears: the physical process of dying, what will happen at the end? Will they suffer? Fear of dying alone, what will happen to spouse or family? It is interesting to note that it is often the fear of dying rather than death itself which predominates. Garfield (1978) lists the following specific fears of the dying:

Table 7.1   Some interventions with emotional responses of the dying

Emotional response	Manifestation	Intervention
Shock	Stunned Hyperactivity/anxiety state Numbness/inactivity	Not to encourage indepen- dence, protect and support, allow to talk
Denial	Acting as if nothing is wrong Obsessive behaviour Looking for second opinions	Do not confront, nor collude with the denial
Anger	Against doctors, NHS, God, family, nurses	Do not get angry back and don't defend people that the patient is angry with
Bargaining	e.g. to live until see daughter married negotiating agreements with God	Allow expression; this can be a very powerful force in the dying
Depression	e.g. with: disablement, loss of control, change in body image, being a burden, loss of relationships and roles, feelings of worthlessness and guilt	Being there Give support Allow patients to be themselves Maintain independence in decision making Respect desire for privacy
Acceptance	Resignation to the inevitable May talk openly about acceptance of dying	Support relatives; this can be particularly difficult for them Help patient learn to live a day at a time Allow expression of fears Maintain hope

- fear of the unknown;
- fear of loneliness;
- fear of sorrow;
- fear of loss of body;
- fear of loss of self-control;
- fear of suffering and pain;
- fear of loss of identity;
- fear of regression.

Exploring with the patient his own personal fears and careful explanation of the dying process can help the patient to cope with such anxiety. Discussion of pain and symptom control and reassurance that he will not die alone unless he specifically requests this can be of great help. Fear of annihilation (end of self) and alienation (loss of relationships with others) are more difficult to work through with patients. Assessing patients' spiritual needs may be important here. Hinton (1967) found that many patients facing death use their faith to find peace and strength. Being able to see other patients having peaceful and dignified deaths and acknowledging and working through their own mourning process can be helpful (some patients arrange their own funeral before death).

Donovan and Girton (1984) outline how the nurse can meet the needs of the dying. They suggest that listening, maintaining hope, using knowledge and identifying patients' strength and resources, allowing patients and relatives to express emotions and describe fears are all part of this. This can be an uncomfortable experience as nurses are forced to listen to things many of us have never had the courage to even think about. It is important to develop skills (such as those outlined in Chapter 4) that encourage the individual to express his feelings, by non-verbal communication (showing an interested expression, eye contact, sitting close to the patient, nodding and making encouraging noises) and verbal communication (use of open-ended questions like 'You seem sad today' or 'This must be very difficult for you right now' to initiate a meaningful conversation, reflecting statements the patient makes, and prompting ('Can you tell me more about that?'). Often strategies as simple as these will open the emotional floodgates and patients will pour out their feelings. Many nurses feel worried about doing this in case they unleash something they cannot handle. This is unlikely; most patients welcome the chance simply to express their feelings and tell their story, and feel relieved afterwards. Robert Buckman's (1988) book on supporting someone who is dying gives very useful advice.

Maintaining hope is an essential component of any helping relationship with the dying. Hope should be identified and translated into a realistic possibility, for example hopes of going home, seeing a beloved pet again, planning a trip. So long as it is not harmful these hopes need not always be totally unreasonable.

Caring for the family

The family should be central to the care of the dying patient and, whenever possible, participate maximally with the patient's care, according to his wishes. This aids anticipatory grieving and can help towards a less stormy bereavement. Many families feel they want to be doing something however small to feel useful. The role of the nurse should therefore be that of facilitator between patient and family rather than the primary caregiver to the exclusion of the family.

The process of grieving for patients is also a process which family members will go through. It is unlikely, however, that they will move through the process at the same rate as the patient. This may be difficult; for instance, in the case where the patient accepts his death before close relatives are ready to, it may seem as if their loved one has turned his back on them and given up. It is also arguable, that as the patient's stresses and suffering diminish as he drifts into a final coma, caregivers and family stresses increase. Lewis (1986), in her review of research into the impact of cancer on the family, has identified the following different sources of stress on the family:

● emotional strain;
● physical demands of caring (e.g. loss of sleep, physical fatigue);
● uncertainty over the patient's health (the fear and anxieties are as great as those of the partner);
● fear of the patient dying;
● altered household roles and lifestyles;
● financial difficulties;
● existential concerns (in one study, 81 per cent of women who stated they had talked with their husbands about his death felt shared expression of dying made it easier to cope with bereavement);
● ways to comfort the patient;
● perceived inadequacy of services;
● sexuality;
● non-convergent needs among household members.

The nurse's role in supporting and facilitating expression of feelings between patients and their families is an essential one. But how can the nurse best help? Freihafer and Felton (1976) asked relatives to rank identified behaviour of carers as helpful and unhelpful.

Helpful behaviour included the following:

● Answer questions honestly.
● Keep patient well groomed and comfortable.
● Calm patient, talk to him, reduce his fear.
● Do not abandon patient.

Unhelpful behaviour included the following:

● Try to get my mind off the patient's condition.
● Cry with me.
● Encourage me to cry.
● Remind me his suffering will soon be over.

As Donovan and Girton (1984) say:

> In the hospital, all family members are outsiders. This fosters frustration – the frustration of helplessly watching a loved one die without being able to do a single thing, while strangers bustle efficiently about doing many things . . . Each person is unique and has unique capabilities. A man can often lift, turn, and move a patient more easily than a woman. He can engage the patient in diversionary

conversation or read to him. A child can help change a bed, draw a picture and give a big hug.

The nurse needs to assess the family's need and desire to be involved continuously and also to assess when it is time for them to have a break to care for their own needs.

Giaquinta (1977), in her work with 100 families living through the death from cancer of a family member, describes ten phases of family functioning within the following four stages:

1. Living with cancer.
2. The living–dying interval.
3. Bereavement.
4. Re-establishment.

During the 'Living with cancer' stage the individual receives an initial diagnosis of cancer and the whole family moves through phases of coping with the impact of the diagnosis. These include functional disruption of usual family roles during illness, treatment and hospitalisation; a search for meaning while the family attempts to gain intellectual mastery over the cancer process; the need to inform others outside the family which can cause feelings of despair, vulnerability and isolation; and displaying emotions. Nurses should aim to foster hope, family cohesion, security courage and problem solving during these phases.

During the living–dying interval the individual ceases to perform familiar roles and is cared for either at home or in hospital. The family must reorganise its roles to cope and lessen the strain. The family also needs time to remember the individual's life history. While this is emotionally painful it is an important phase to go through for both patient and family. Through the use of pictures, scrapbooks and family albums the nurse may facilitate this process.

Bereavement coincides with the imminent death of the individual. Separation and mourning are the tasks of the family at this stage. Nursing interventions here should be towards promoting intimacy between family members and fostering relief through the expression of grief.

Re-establishment signals the end of mourning when the family may re-enter their social environment which extends beyond the family.

Dealing with a death on the ward

Until now, the discussion has centred on coping with the needs of the dying patient and his family. But what about once the patient actually dies? Many nurses will be faced with dealing with this for the first time once they are qualified and may be on their own in charge of the ward at the time.

The flow diagram in Fig. 7.8 includes information relating to the responsibilities of the nurse in charge of the ward at the time of death. This is really just a memory aid to help the nurse through the experience. Each hospital or health authority is likely to have its own policies and procedures regarding last offices, and where and when relatives can collect patients' property and the death certificates. It is therefore recommended that local information be consulted regarding these.

Guide to last offices

Hospital policies regarding last offices should be referred to, but the main principle is to straighten the body and make it presentable. Some nurses feel that since it is the last thing they will do for the patient, it is important to wash the patient, applying nice smelling talcs, and make the patient look as clean and peaceful as possible. This is not necessarily a must unless the body is particularly dirty with leaking fluids; often the body is washed anyway in the mortuary and by the undertakers. But if there is plenty of time, and especially if the relative wish to view the body, this may seem important. It is also necessary to bear in mind different cultural and religious practices regarding last offices (see Table 7.2).

Conclusion

Caring for the dying presents immense challenges to nurses, particularly in busy, acute hospital wards. The memory of the way a close relative was cared for in their last days or hours can stay with the bereaved person for many years and if the event was badly handled or traumatic, can add to his burden of grief. This means that for nurses dealing with both the dying individual and his family there is little room for error or making good clumsy handling of such delicate and painful events.

This chapter has tried to provide an introduction to the physical and psychological care of the dying and to offer suggestions regarding important areas of such care. The emotional toll caring for dying patients and their families can place on nurses and other professionals is very great. The importance of seeking out colleagues or friends who can share these emotions cannot be underestimated and is vital to personal survival and health.

Fig. 7.8   Dealing with a death on the ward (Source: Jessica Corner 1988)

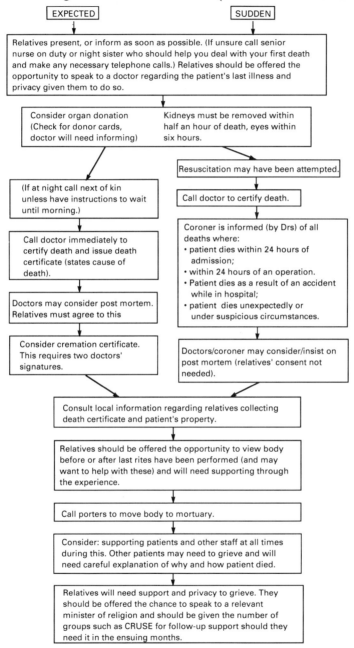

EXPECTED   SUDDEN

Relatives present, or inform as soon as possible. (If unsure call senior nurse on duty or night sister who should help you deal with your first death and make any necessary telephone calls.) Relatives should be offered the opportunity to speak to a doctor regarding the patient's last illness and privacy given them to do so.

Consider organ donation (Check for donor cards, doctor will need informing) — Kidneys must be removed within half an hour of death, eyes within six hours.

Resuscitation may have been attempted.

(If at night call next of kin unless have instructions to wait until morning.)

Call doctor to certify death.

Call doctor immediately to certify death and issue death certificate (states cause of death).

Coroner is informed (by Drs) of all deaths where:
• patient dies within 24 hours of admission;
• within 24 hours of an operation.
• Patient dies as a result of an accident while in hospital;
• patient dies unexpectedly or under suspicious circumstances.

Doctors may consider post mortem. Relatives must agree to this

Consider cremation certificate. This requires two doctors' signatures.

Doctors/coroner may consider/insist on post mortem (relatives' consent not needed).

Consult local information regarding relatives collecting death certificate and patient's property.

Relatives should be offered the opportunity to view body before or after last rites have been performed (and may want to help with these) and will need supporting through the experience.

Call porters to move body to mortuary.

Consider: supporting patients and other staff at all times during this. Other patients may need to grieve and will need careful explanation of why and how patient died.

Relatives will need support and privacy to grieve. They should be offered the chance to speak to a relevant minister of religion and should be given the number of groups such as CRUSE for follow-up support should they need it in the ensuing months.

Recommended reading (and also for Relatives) :
DHSS Leaflet *What to do after a death* D49/October 1987 which can be obtained from: DHSS Leaflets unit, P.o. Box 21, Stanmore, Middlesex HA7 1AY

Table 7.2 Notes on caring for dying patients of different religions (after Neuberger 1987)

Religion	Food restrictions	Other practices	Attitudes towards death	What to do with body	Other last rites information
Judaism	Kosher diet		Differing views on the after life Emphasis is on the here and now	Leave body for 8 minutes. Straighten limbs and tie jaw, by family if available. Body is not left alone until the Sexton (Jewish undertaker) removes it	None May request Rabbi before death Important to differentiate between orthodox, liberal reform jews
Hinduism	No beef Often vegetarian May have own food while in hospital	Hindu women – modesty is very important. Often reluctant to undress for examination Total privacy for bed bathing essential Bath by member of same sex Conversation about pain and problems with genito-urinary systems or bowels is taboo particularly if spouse is present		Sometimes will lay body on floor and surround with candles Post mortem is disrespectful and is objected to	Cremation Hindu priest will be helpful and will help the patient deal philosophically with death
Sikism	Often vegetarian, including not eating eggs Few eat beef No alcohol		Reincarnation	In consultation with family, close eyes, straighten body, wrap in plain sheet	Family wash and dress body Cremation is normal and within 24 hours if possible Women wear white as a symbol of mourning

Table 7.2 (contd.)

Religion	Food restrictions	Other practices	Attitudes towards death	What to do with body	Other last rites information
Islam	Vegetarian unless Halal meat is available	Modesty is crucial Women fully clothed at all times, even at night Women may object to male doctors and nurses	Believe in after life	Body should not be touched by non-Moslem. If essential wear gloves to prevent contact. If family willing close eyes, straighten limbs, head turned towards Mecca. Body placed in plain sheet unwashed	Family members perform last rites. Should sit or lie with face turned to Mecca whilst dying, while another Moslem whispers prayers into their ear. Buried, never cremated, usually within 24 hours
Buddhism	Often vegetarian	Strict rules of hygiene. Wash before meditation, after defaecation and before medication. May refuse pain relief			

References

Birch, J. (1983) 'Anxiety and conflict in nurse education', in Davis, B. (ed.) *Research into Nurse Education*, London: Croom Helm.

Bowlby, J. (1961) 'Processes of mourning', *International Journal of Psychoanalysis*, Vol. 42, No. 4, pp. 317–40.

Buckman, R. (1988) *I Don't Know What To Say: How to help and support someone who is dying*, London: Papermac.

Carr, A. T. (1982) Dying and bereavement, in Halty, J. (ed.) *Psychology for Health Professionals*, Basingstoke: Macmillan Press.

Donovan, N. I. and Girton, S. E. (1984) *Cancer Care Nursing*, Norwalk, Connecticut: Appleton Century Crofts.

Drummond-Mills, W. (1983) *Problems Related to the Nursing Management of the Dying Patient*, Unpublished MSc Thesis, University of Glasgow.

Freihafer, P. and Felton, G. (1976) 'Nursing behaviours in bereavement: An explanatory study', *Nursing Research*, Vol. 25, pp. 332–7.

Fulton, R. (1976) *Death and Identity*, Charles Press Inc.

Garfield, C. A. (1978) *Psychosocial Care of the Dying Patient*, New York: McGraw Hill Book Company.

Giaquinta, B. (1977) 'Helping families face the crisis of cancer', *American Journal of Nursing*, October 1977, pp. 1585–9.

Glaser, B. G. and Strauss, A. L. (1965) *Awareness of Dying*, Chicago: Aldine.

Glaser, B. G. and Strauss, A. L. (1968) *Time for Dying*, Chicago: Aldine.

Hanks, G. W. (1983) 'Management of symptoms in advanced cancer', *Update*, 15 May, pp. 1691–1702.

Hanks, G. W. (1985) 'The management of pain in advanced cancer', in Wilkes, E. (ed.) *Terminal Care*, Update Postgraduate Series, Napp Laboratories Ltd.

Hinton, J. (1967) *Dying*, London: Pelican Books.

Hunt, J. N. (1977) 'Patients with protracted pain: a survey conducted at the London Hospital', *Journal of Medical Ethics*, Vol. 3, pp. 61–73.

Knight, M. and Field, D. (1981) 'A silent conspiracy: coping with dying cancer patients on an acute surgical ward', *Journal of Advanced Nursing*, Vol. 6, pp. 221–9.

Kubler Ross, E. (1969) *On Death and Dying*, New York: Macmillan.

Lathlean, J., Smith, G. and Bradley, S. (1986) *Post Registration Development Schemes Evaluation*. King's College, University of London.

Lewis, F. M. (1986) 'The impact of cancer on the family: a critical analysis of the research literature', *Patient Education and Counselling*, pp. 269–89.

Lindemann, E. (1944) 'Symptomatology and management of acute grief', *American Journal of Psychiatry*, Vol. 101, pp. 141–8.

McCaffery, M. (1979) *Nursing the patient in pain*. Adapted for the UK by Soffaer, B. Lippincott Nursing Series, London: Harper and Row.

Neuberger, J. (1987) *Caring for Dying People of Different Faiths*, London: Austen Cornish Pubs.

Parkes, C. M. (1972) *Bereavement Studies of Grief in Adult Life*, London: Pelican Books.

arkes, C. M. (1978) 'Home or hospital? Terminal care as seen by surviving spouses', *Journal of the Royal College of General Practitioners*, Vol. 28, pp. 19–30.

arkes, C. M. and Parkes, J. (1984) 'Hospice versus hospital care – re-evaluation after 10 years as seen by surviving spouses', *Postgraduate Medical Journal*, February.

uint, J. C. (1965) 'Institutionalised practices of information control', *Psychiatry*, Vol. 28, No. 2, pp. 119–132.

uint, J. C. (1967) *The Nurse and the Dying Patient*, New York: Macmillan.

aylor, H. (1983) *The Hospice Movement in Britain: Its Role and Future*, Centre for Policy on Ageing Report.

wycross, R. G. and Lack, S. A. (1983) *Symptom Control in Far Advanced Cancer: Pain Relief*, London: Pitman.

wycross, R. G. and Lack, S. A. (1984) *Therapeutics in Terminal Cancer*, Edinburgh: Churchill Livingstone.

alker, V. A. and Dicks, B. (1987) 'Pain assessment charts in the management of chronic cancer pain', *Palliative Medicine*, Vol. 1, pp.111–6.

ebster, N. E. (1981) 'Communicating with dying patients', *Nursing Times*, 4 June, pp. 999–1002.

ertheimer, A. (1986) 'A rotten way to die', Society Tomorrow, *The Guardian*. Wednesday 1 September, p. 11.

urther reading

sychosocial care of the dying

tle	Author/publisher	Comments
n Death and Dying	E. Kubler Ross, Tavistock (1969)	Useful book on Kubler Ross's work on emotional reactions to dying. Paperback.
ying	John Hinton, Pelican (1967)	Inexpensive paperback looking at aspects of terminal illness.
ealing with Death and ying: a New Nursing illbook.	Urosevich P. R., 2nd edn, Spring House Corporation (1984)	Useful, easy to read text with study notes and guidelines on all aspects of caring for the dying.
aring for Dying People of ifferent Faiths*	Julia Neuberger, The Lisa Sainsbury Foundation Series (1987), Austen Cornish Pubs.	Useful inexpensive book on cultural aspects of dying.
Don't Know What to Say. ow to Help and Support meone Who is Dying*	Dr Robert Buckman, Papermac (1988)	Very helpful text, with advice on supporting the dying.

Highly recommended.

Symptom control

Title	Author/publisher	Comments
Nursing Care of the Dying Patient	Alison Charles Edwards, Beaconsfield (1983)	Useful nursing text on all aspects of care of the dying
*Nursing the Patient in Pain**	Margo McCaffery, adapted for the UK by Beatrice Soffaer. Lippincott Nursing Series, Harper & Row (1979)	Excellent text on caring for the patient in pain. Particularly chapter on assessment and non-pharmacological interventions in pain control.
*Pain: Clinical Manual for Nursing Practice**	Margo McCaffery, C. V. Mosby (1989)	As above.
Cancer Pain Relief	World Health Organisation. Geneva (1986).	WHO guidelines for Cancer Pain Relief. Booklet. From bookseller or from HMSO Useful and easy to read.
Therapeutics in Terminal Care	Twycross, R. and Lack, S. A., Churchill Livingstone (1984)	Useful, pharmacological reference book to the complex area of prescribing in pain and symptom control. Aimed at doctors (useful as ward reference book).
*A Guide to Symptom Relief in Advanced Cancer**	Regnard, C. and Davies, A., Haigh & Hockland (1986)	Excellent quick reference booklet to symptom control useful in all dying patients
Oral Morphine in Advanced Cancer	Twycross, R. and Lack, S., Beaconsfield (1984)	Booklet written in question and answer format which makes it easy to read.
Hospice Care Principles and Practice	Corr, C. A., and Corr, D. M., Faber (1983)	Inexpensive collection of essays on terminal care.

*Highly recommended.

8 Change in Nursing

RICHARD MCMAHON

Introduction

Nursing is going through a period of rapid change and development, spurred on by stimuli from both internal and external sources. From within the profession, nurses are increasingly questioning current practice and demanding higher standards of care. Nurse researchers and educationalists are broadening the understanding of nurses and nursing, whilst the official and unofficial leaders in nursing are pressing for the adoption of new ideas. External influences such as the demographic changes resulting in fewer school leavers entering nursing, and the increase in the number of elderly people in the country are making a major impact on nursing. Political decisions affecting the management of community health services, relatively newly identified health problems such as AIDS, the greater sophistication and spread of technology in medicine and many other factors all have potential for influencing the way that nurses practice.

Change is an inevitable challenge to the newly qualified nurse. Change has the potential to be stimulating and rewarding. However, if it is badly managed it can cause resentment and dissatisfaction. The purpose of this chapter is to help the newly qualified nurse to understand and cope with change and to gain knowledge about initiating change herself. Frequently the newly registered nurse is not the generator of change herself, but as a trained nurse she can be an invaluable supporter of new ideas and practices. Unfortunately, this can, on occasion, lead to potential conflict with colleagues. It is important for the nurse to recognise the efforts of others to introduce change and to consider how she can deal with her own and others' feelings towards that change.

First, it is useful to explore the process of change and some problems that may be encountered in coping with, or implementing change. Then, within this context, some of the major changes affecting nursing practice and education are considered, and finally, ways in which nurses can keep up to date with developments are outlined.

Understanding change in nursing

The nature of change

Change has been defined as: 'any planned or unplanned alteration of the status quo in an organism, situation or process' Lippitt (1973).

Planning and handling change requires knowledge, skill and an understanding and ability to empathise with people. There have been problems in this respect in nursing. For example, in many areas when an attempt was first made to introduce the nursing process, ward sisters were told to change – in some cases overnight. The ensuing failure of the nursing process to function, the resentment amongst staff and the frustration experienced by those trying to promote change can be easily imagined. Change through the exercising of physical or social power is less likely to gain acceptance than a strategy which aims to re-educate and influence the attitudes of those involved. Similarly, if the people involved in changing can appreciate a benefit for themselves in adopting the new idea, then again the chances of success are greatly improved. Where power is exerted to alter a situation, the participation of those on the receiving end is not necessary. However, by contrast, if power is not used, participation in the change process of all involved is a major strategy for achieving change.

Hersey and Blanchard (1977) suggest a hierarchy of difficulty and time involved in changing people (see Fig. 8.1). For example, if the aim is to change eating habits in an elderly person, it could be relatively easy to teach that person so that he or she understands that brown bread contains more fibre than white bread. However, that individual might have the attitude that brown bread is for the poor – remembering that to be the case when he or she was younger. But even if the nurse could change that attitude, the old person might still *prefer* white bread and hence not show any change in behaviour. Clearly, the time and effort involved in persuading that individual to change would be multiplied if the nurse was trying to change a group of elderly people, each with different knowledge, attitudes and behaviour.

Fig. 8.1   A hierarchy of difficulty and time involved in changing people (Note: a change in a lower element in the hierarchy does not necessarily lead to a change in the next element) (Adapted from Hersey and Blanchard 1977)

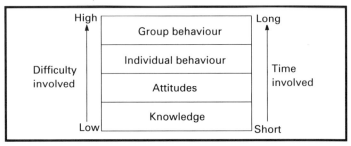

One of the ways that change occurs is through the efforts of a 'change agent'. Mauksch and Miller (1981) identify two types of change agent, formal and informal. Formal change agents have had their role legitimised by the institution in which they find themselves. Informal change agents try to create change out of their own motivation, but are rarely in a position of authority and hence have to rely on persuasion to achieve their objectives. This is frequently the situation of the newly qualified staff nurse who finds herself wishing to change the area in which she is working, based on the education and experience she gained during her training. However, she has no authority to order or encourage change in the ward sister or other members of staff who have been in that area for a far greater time.

Change agents may also be internal or external: that is, within the system or area in which change is desired (e.g. the ward sister or staff nurse in the case of a ward) or outside it, such as the nursing officer or clinical nurse manager. When the nursing process was being implemented, many health authorities employed 'nursing process co-ordinators' to stimulate the change to that approach. These external change agents had no authority as they were outside the management hierarchy, and consequently these nurses had to rely on their abilities to create change without exerting power.

Change, then, is a complicated process, the catalyst for which is normally an individual or change agent. The way nurses can succeed in planning and implementing change needs further description.

The newly qualified nurse as change agent

Nurses who have recently completed their training nearly always find themselves in the role of internal and informal change agents. Although such nurses rarely have much formal authority to create change, by bringing a fresh mind to a situation they can often see through the dogmatic approach which may be taken by others.

Ottoway (1982) suggested that change agents can be further divided into three types, all of which are necessary and valuable.

Change generators

In general, these are people who identify issues and bring them to the attention of others. They could be charismatic leaders in nursing, influential at a local level, or external to the health care system altogether. Change generators tend to be independent and resourceful people who are willing to be criticised by others for their beliefs.

Perhaps surprisingly, it can be argued that the recently qualified nurse can act as a change generator. For example, a nurse who has recently completed her training may have new ideas for supervising the experience of students on the ward based on her own up-to-date experience. In some cases this type of nurse will be offered a job by a senior nurse in an attempt to move forward a ward which has been particularly resistant to implementing new ideas. This is not an enviable situation for any nurse, and unless that nurse has great strength and initiative she may well either conform to the norms already established on the ward or become disenchanted and leave. However, where there is an environment in which new ideas are encouraged, or at least not suppressed, the newly registered nurse can provide ideas and act as a stimulus for those with the authority and ability to initiate change.

Change implementers

These nurses are people who respond to the need for change fostered by the change generators. In a ward setting the ward sister is potentially a powerful change implementer, with those lower in the hierarchy often creating change through the ward sister. Nurses who are unable to do this must avoid a situation where they implement change unilaterally when they are 'in charge'. If this occurs, care may end up being delivered one way when that nurse is on duty and in a different way when the ward sister is present. This causes confusion for patients and other nurses, fails to address the underlying problem, and does not lead to lasting change.

One of the ways in which a staff nurse can implement change in an area where there is resistance to innovation is through taking on responsibility for a small project herself. For example, she might wish to introduce a rack of health education leaflets relevant to the type of patients most commonly admitted to the ward. The steps of the change process will be described in greater detail later, but it is obvious that the nurse will have to consider the time involved in writing to organisations for the leaflets, the cost of the rack, the responsibility for stocking and tidying the rack and the storage of back-up supplies of leaflets. Once she has established some ideas for solutions to these issues she can then approach the sister and other staff with her proposal. Where it is deemed to be a good idea, with obvious benefits for patients, and especially when it is unlikely to create much extra work for anyone other than the person making the proposal, there is a good chance that it will be accepted. Having gained agreement, the nurse must see the project through, and later judge whether it has succeeded. By gaining the co-operation of a colleague it is possible to spread the responsibility, share the work involved and be mutually supportive. There is also more chance that the innovation, or activity, will continue even when the nurse is absent or has left the post.

Change adopters

By taking the role of a change adopter the new staff nurse can make an enormously valuable contribution to promoting innovation in nursing. The forward-thinking ward sister will seek the reactions and opinions of her staff prior to introducing change. When approached, the staff nurse may find herself responding to a new idea in a number of ways.

First, she can express her approval or disapproval of the idea in principle. A desire to provide the answer the staff nurse thinks the sister wants to hear should be resisted since it may result in an 'easier life' initially but can cause longer term resentment and frustration. Strong feelings should be explored and where the nurse has insufficient knowledge to form an opinion she should admit to this. Sometimes it is only after some thought that a considered opinion can be arrived at, in which case the nurse should seek an opportunity to discuss the idea further with the sister.

Second, she can express her views or reservations for implementing the innovation in practice, thus opening the way for more discussion or, third, if she is already relatively satisfied about the ideas, she can offer her support to them and to their implementation should that occur.

By her own thoughtful approach to the change, the staff nurse can carry others with her. She can help those with worries about the change who may be unwilling to challenge the sister and provide an example and enthusiasm for the innovation. This kind of support is encouraging and necessary for the ward sister who should also appreciate constructive criticism and forewarning of problems arising out of the change.

The change process

Several people have tried to identify the steps that must be completed if change is to be successful. The newly qualified nurse is unlikely to find herself in a situation where she will be expected to implement change on a large scale, such as developing primary nursing on a ward, but if she is aware of the process of change she can contribute more effectively to it.

One way in which the stages of the change process may be described is shown in Fig. 8.2. Clearly, change should be planned, otherwise the likelihood of resistance and unwanted side-effects is great. Resistance is likely to be less if all those involved in the change have been consulted and involved in the change process. If the change agent can engender the need for change in the staff, then often they can then come up their own solutions if they are provided with sufficient information.

The person planning the change cannot do so until she has a good understanding of the working relationships in the area. Furthermore, ideally, the staff need to know the person who will implement the change. There should be a relationship based on trust between the individuals or within the group, with this trust being built on good communication. By understanding the social environment in which she is working, the nurse is able to identify the unofficial

Fig. 8.2   The steps of the change process

1. Recognising and analysing the problem.
2. Assessing motivation, capacity and resources for change.
3. Assessing change agent's own motivation and resources.
4. Identifying the goal.
5. Planning strategy for change and identifying progressive objectives.
6. Implementing and supporting change.
7. Maintaining change and setting up self-supporting mechanisms.
8. Evaluating change.
9. Terminating the relationship.

'leaders' of opinion, who, if they can be won over, will influence the opinions of several other nurses.

   The initiator of change cannot work unsupported for long. The identification of a person with similar values and attitudes who can listen sympathetically to the frustrations of creating change is essential for the continued motivation of the change agent. This could be a tutor, a senior nurse or a nurse from another ward. Where a number of nurses are working as change agents in isolation, coming together in a support group may be useful for some people (Heineken and Nussbaumer 1976).

   Example 8.1 illustrates how the framework provided in Fig. 8.2 can be used to work through a problem and make change. Like the problem-oriented nursing process, this framework for planning change starts with the gathering of as much data as possible to clarify the problem, and proposing and testing different solutions, based on the resources available not only for the change but also within the change agent. The choosing of the strategies to be adopted and the setting of objectives is followed by the implementation of the change. Change agents should work for their own redundancy and set up the system in such a way that it is not dependent on an individual for its continuation. Once the new norm is self-supporting the success of the change can be evaluated and the unexpected effects dealt with. Finally, at some stage the change agent must withdraw and leave the system to continue in her absence.

Resistance to change

Resistance to change is almost bound to occur where change of any significance is planned. The degree of resistance relies on a number of factors. First, the magnitude of the change – minor adjustments to a system are less likely to meet with disapproval than the removal of one system and the introduction of a new one. Second is the degree to which the change affects the values and attitudes of the individuals involved. A plan to abolish nurses' caps in a long-established

Example 8.1   Using the change process to solve problems about visiting times

Newly qualified nurses can be particularly sensitive to problems on the ward that more experienced nurses may overlook through familiarity. One such problem is the difficulty experienced by some relatives in visiting during specified visiting hours. The change process can be used to think through the stages that might be appropriate for exploring the problem and improving the situation.

Having identified the problem, the nurse can question the basis on which visiting times have originated. The nurse then moves naturally to the second step of the process – that of assessing the potential and motivation amongst her colleagues for a change to the system. Exploring the issues in informal discussion with the ward sister and other nurses can help the nurse to ascertain the extent of the support and resistance she might experience. Following this analysis, the staff nurse would need to examine her own motivation and energy to see through the change.

At this stage the goals should be identified. In this case the more general goal might be the greater satisfaction of patients and their relatives with the system for visiting, and the more specific aim could be the decrease in complaints from patients' relatives about the hours.

The nurse's strategy for change would then be planned. This might consist of the following. First, other nurses need to be made more aware of the problem by talking with them and highlighting individual patients whose relatives cannot visit during the allotted times. Second, the staff nurse knows the character of the sister and her amenability to change. She might decide not to suggest a solution to the sister, merely to pose the question: 'How can we help these visitors?'. Third, she could ask that visiting times be put on the agenda for the next ward meeting. Prior to the meeting she could ensure that one or more of her colleagues who supports change in the system can be present at the meeting; change put forward by a group is often more effective than a lone voice.

The progressive goal could be to obtain agreement for alteration in the ward policy for initiatives on a trial basis, whereas the immediate action might be to concentrate on this as one example whereby set visiting times are abolished for an experimental period. A number of important factors need consideration before change can be implemented. For example, the sister may require various other people to be informed (or even involved) before proceeding (e.g. the senior nurse who is responsible for the unit) and the effects of any attempts in other parts of the hospital to change visiting hours should be studied. The outcomes of the new system can be monitored, for example by systematically recording the perceptions of patients, their relatives and ward staff. The staff nurse can play a major part in the evaluation and, at the end of the trial period, the advantages and disadvantages can be weighed up. If it is decided to adopt the change, new signs for the ward regarding visiting hours can be ordered and a relative permanence assumed.

hospital will be treated as trivial by some but as a major affront by others. Third, it is considered to be generally true that people fear the unknown, and it follows that people will resist what they fear. Two-way communication is a prerequisite to successful change. Those involved must not only have information, but should also have ample opportunity to voice fears and reservations. To do this honestly, those involved in the change must respect and trust the person suggesting the change. Fourth, nurses are unlikely to support schemes which disadvantage either their financial or social standing unless the benefits are perceived to outweigh these factors. Finally, the nurse initiating change must not forget that some nurses will resist out of the security achieved through maintaining the status quo, whilst others will have seriously considered the change proposed and decided that they should not support it.

Resistance to change manifests itself in many ways. It is sometimes easier to deal with the resister who is voluble in her resistance, as she will clearly make her objections known. In contrast, the person who says that she understands and agrees with the change, yet does not show this in her actions can initially be difficult to identify. People reacting this way need to be confronted with the lack of unity between their words and deeds in a manner aimed at helping rather than criticising the individual.

In summary, all change should be carefully planned and it is essential that those participating in the change are consulted and involved in the process. Resistance to change is common and can lead to self-doubt and pessimism for the person initiating the change. The newly qualified staff nurse can play a crucial part in creating change. She can generate change by providing ideas and information for others. She can implement change herself, or support the efforts of her colleagues who may be attempting to implement change themselves.

Current innovations in nursing

There are a number of major documents and policies influencing nursing practice and education, including governmental White Papers such as the NHS review, *Working for Patients* (DoH 1989a), and for community care, *Caring for People* (DoH 1989b), and national initiatives such as the reform of initial nurse education by Project 2000 (UKCC 1986), the proposals for post-registration education and practice (UKCC 1990), known as PREPP, and the implementation of the clinical grading scheme. Although the newly registered nurse may not feel that she is affected directly by all of these, at the very least, the ethos of the organisations within which nurses work is influenced by such changes. Further, Project 2000 is resulting in different demands for trained nurses and the introduction of new roles within nursing, the Post-Registration Education and Practice Project (PREPP) project is aimed at providing a review system and a personal professional development 'profile' for all registered nurses, and clinical grading automatically encompasses all qualified nurses to senior nurse level.

The reform of the NHS

Since its inception in 1948, the National Health Service has been the subject of many government reports and has undergone multiple reorganisations. These have frequently addressed issues relating to the structure of the Service, the most recent of these being the review of the NHS, resulting in the White Paper entitled *Working for Patients* (DoH 1989a). The White Paper has three central aims designed to raise the standard of service to patients without incurring undue additional long-term financial support, namely:

1. extending patient choice;
2. delegating responsibility to those best placed to respond to the needs of patients;
3. securing the best value for money.

The proposals in this document allow major acute hospitals to become 'self-governing' and may lead to the newly qualified nurse finding herself working in a hospital which is managing its own affairs rather than being under the direction of the local district health authority. In this situation, the hospital will operate as an NHS trust, earning much of its revenue from the services it provides under contracts from the health authorities, general practitioners and the private sector. One of the implications of this for nurses in these hospitals is that their pay will no longer be nationally negotiated, with the directors of a trust deciding both the level of pay and the conditions of employment. This may be advantageous or disadvantageous for the nurse, as pay is likely to be linked with the profitability of specialisms (*Nursing Times* 1989).

In addition, the way the service is financed is to be altered, resulting in a strengthened role for the regional health authorities and the district health authorities (DHAs) having to buy the best services they can from their own hospitals, other DHA hospitals, self-governing hospitals or the private sector. Also, the White Paper proposes a major extension of the system, called 'resource management', a project introduced by the NHS Management Board in 1986. (Millar, 1989, provides a helpful guide to how it works and what it means for nursing practice.) Nurses in six hospitals around England have taken part in pilot schemes for the government's Resource Management Initiative (RMI). For example, the Freeman Hospital began by taking a patient's medical record as a starting point for looking at how resources are managed, and has gone on to refine a nursing manpower information system as one part of its resource management project. This computerised system, developed from a program written by Jean Ball, known as *Criteria for Care*, entails activity analysis, and, in collaboration with the patients, assessing patient dependency and monitoring the quality of nursing care given. The implementation of this system and the implications for the nurses involved are described by Vousden (1989).

Initiatives have, however, been operating in hospitals without the support of the RMI project. For example, in 1986 the Radcliffe Infirmary, Oxford, started a trial when ward sisters demanded to be allowed to manage their resources and control their own budgets. Their work has been based on the belief that 'decisions regarding patient care and the authority over resources to provide that care should be made as near to the bedside as possible' (Chalmers 1990). Thus the Oxford Nurse Management System has been developed to determine the demand (patient need), the supply (nursing hours planned and available to meet the need), and the cost of nursing care for each patient (Wood 1990). The White Paper has given further impetus to such initiatives, and has stimulated the implementation of clinical management whereby the budget for a unit, such as a group of wards, will be managed by a team consisting of a nurse, an administrator and a doctor. This is likely to result in nurses at ward level having to justify their nursing establishment or need for equipment on a recurring basis, rather than having an automatic budgetary increase each year.

This White Paper and the one on Community Care are the subject of the NHS and Community Care Bill, passing through parliament during 1990, and the results of the Bill are likely to be implemented from 1 April 1991.

The reform of nurse education

In 1986, the United Kingdom Central Council for Nursing, Midwifery and Health Visiting published proposals for major reform of initial nurse education in Britain (UKCC 1986). 'Project 2000' – as it is known – proposed that nurse education should have close links with higher education, with learners taking on supernumerary status and receiving grants or bursaries rather than salaries. It pointed out the 'complex and varied pattern of education and training leading to 10 different parts of the register' (UKCC 1987) and outlined a future three-year preparation, beginning with a Common Foundation Programme (subsequently agreed to last for eighteen months), followed by a 'branch' programme in nursing care of the adult, the child, the mentally handicapped person and in mental health. Alongside the proposed changes in registered nurse education, the UKCC suggested that nursing should have a grade of support worker, and also that the training of enrolled nurses should cease.

Following a major consultation exercise the document was generally well received, although the RCN urged the UKCC to reconsider its recommendations regarding the location of the base for nurse education. The RCN consulted its membership and suggested that nurse education should be based in higher education rather than merely working in close liaison with outside colleges, polytechnics and universities (RCN 1986). The process of agreeing change was by no means easy, as highlighted by a research study conducted by Lathlean (1989) to identify how policies were made to rationalise the organisation of nurse education at this time. Project 2000 was accepted by the government in May 1988 with few alterations or conditions, except that a service contribution of 20 per cent was considered appropriate. One item the government did focus on, however, was the possible shortage of nurses arising out of terminating enrolled nurse training. In return for this the government asked for the 'entry gate' into nurse training to be widened. Similarly it asked for clarification of the nature and role of the new support worker, now called health care assistants.

The introduction of Project 2000 programmes is being phased, and several schemes are underway. Inevitably, there will be problems with such a major change, and certainly in the transition period one of the major difficulties experienced has been that of running two systems of education alongside each other.

For nurses who trained under the old system the new route to registration taken by learners means appreciating the new values inherent in the system (see Fig. 8.3). Although the students will not spend appreciably less time on the wards than previously, the qualified staff on the ward must recognise that students will not be there as part of the workforce. Instead, they are likely to be working alongside expert practitioners in an environment which, whilst being practice orientated, will cater for the needs of those learning to practise. The students may well bring attitudes and approaches to practice based on a framework very different to the medical model under which most current qualified nurses trained. Furthermore, the proportion of students without experience of life beyond health care is likely to shrink quite considerably, with learners bringing a great deal of experience and knowledge of outside issues. The changes in nurse education have implications not only for the nurses of the future, but also for those qualifying now, as the success of the new approach will rely on efforts by all those who will come into contact with the new students.

Nurses who have trained under the old system may wonder if they will be disadvantaged in relation to those training under the new system. For example, the National Boards are requiring Project 2000 courses to reach at least Diploma level 2, and the courses will provide credits towards a General or Honours Degree or points under the Credit Accumulation Transfer Scheme (CATS) (see Chapter 9 for further detail of the CATS scheme). However, greater attention is being paid to post-registration training for staff, in particular through PREPP, and this should help not only to develop the skills of traditionally trained nurses, but also to provide opportunities for those who

Fig. 8.3   One way the new route to registration may look following the implementation of Project 2000

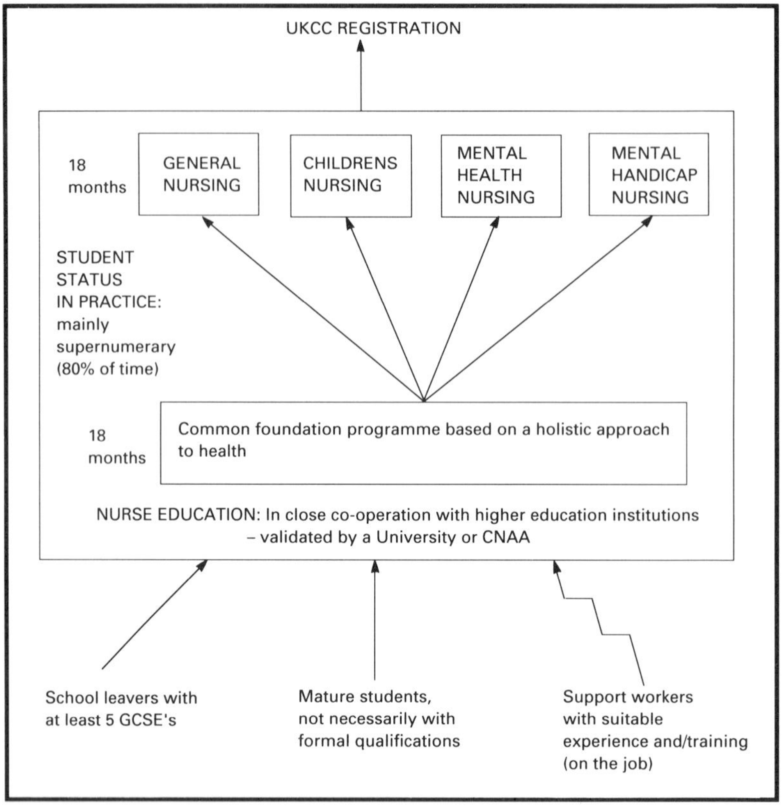

also wish to gain credits towards further qualifications. Chapter 9 explores some of these opportunities and considers the implications of PREPP.

Clinical grading for nurses

The pay structure for clinical nurses has also been the subject of change and controversy. Whereas in the past enrolled nurses, staff nurses and most ward sisters and charge nurses have been on the same incremental ladder as others with the same job title, now nurses are graded on the job they do, rather than the job title. Therefore, the newly registered nurse who is rarely in charge of the ward will be on a different incremental ladder to a nurse who regularly takes that responsibility. This system allows for some negotiation about grading where the nurse finds that the job in reality does not correspond with the job description and allotted grade.

The organisation of nursing care

The way in which nursing is organised on a ward has been the subject of change, particularly in the last two decades. Traditionally, ward nursing was managed on the basis of a hierarchy. It was the role of the sister and staff nurses to direct the care given to patients by learners and unqualified staff. This led to some problems. In many instances, care was fragmented, and increasingly the division of labour on the ward was such that the trained nurses performed managerial, technical and medically related tasks, whilst the untrained staff took on the less valued aspects of care such as bathing, feeding, exercising and talking to patients. In the late 1970s the nursing process brought with it a re-examination of values, with a recognition that care should be based on the individuality of patients and that the nurse–patient relationship was something to be treasured and nurtured.

Individualised care under the guise of the nursing process has been demonstrated to benefit patients (Miller 1988), though the way the concepts were implemented led to a number of limitations. For example, although patient allocation and the systematic approach of the nursing process resulted in a certain degree of continuity of individualised care, this was limited as nurses rarely cared for the same group of patients for more than a few consecutive shifts. Also, wards still operated on the basis of a hierarchy with accountability for care hardly ever being vested in the person actually caring for the patient. This resulted in some patients receiving care almost exclusively from unqualified nurses during a shift. To overcome these problems many areas have chosen a new approach to the organisation of nursing work known as *primary nursing*.

The system of primary nursing – clearly an important development in nursing – has already been described at length in Chapter 2 and referred to in Chapters 3 and 4. Primary nursing was developed in Minnesota, USA, and most of the early research has been American. Unfortunately, much of this has been criticised as being descriptive or anecdotal (Tutton and Ersser 1991), and there are relatively few British studies. For example, there has been a study of the implementation of primary nursing in two nursing developments in the early 1980s (Pearson 1988), and another that compared relations among nurses on primary and non-primary nursing wards and found that the emphasis on the former was on collegiality and collaboration and in the latter, on hierarchy and direction of actions from the top (McMahon 1990). A comprehensive descriptive and theoretical account of the theory and practice of primary nursing in the United Kingdom can be found in Ersser and Tutton (1991).

The introduction of new roles

An inevitable part of change is the introduction of new roles or the variation of existing ones. For example, primary nursing affects the jobs of both the staff nurse and the sister and, in some instances, the original posts cease to exist or at least are different in their nature (this is discussed further in Chapter 3). Examples of new roles include nurse practitioners, in essence nurses with the autonomy to admit and discharge patients to and from the primary health care system, and lecturer practitioners who are nurses with responsibilities spanning practice and education.

Nurse practitioners

A new move in the community has been the development of the role of 'nurse practitioner'. This has been highlighted by the Community Nursing Review (DHSS 1986) which recommended that the principle be adopted of introducing the nurse practitioner into primary health care. In this country nurse practitioners have worked in a complementary way with general practitioners, providing an alternative service for people with health problems outside the hospital setting.

Originally a nurse practitioner scheme was developed in the early 1960s in Colorado to provide care for children. There was a shortage of medical staff in the United States at that time, and although this did not give the impetus for the development, it did provide an opportunity which nurses recognised and grasped (Silver *et al.* 1985). Nurses were trained in many of the examination and diagnostic skills of doctors. However, the purpose of the project was not to develop 'nurse doctors' but to train nurses to be able to give a high standard of care based on concepts of health and prevention, and to be highly skilled, research-based, accountable and autonomous. Since those early days, nurse practitioners have spread into many different fields of health care in many different settings.

In Britain, Barbara Stilwell offered the services of a nurse practitioner alongside the doctors in a Birmingham health centre. Like the doctors, Stilwell was able to perform a physical examination of her patient, and also prescribed a limited number of drugs. Unlike the general practitioners she could offer appointments lasting twenty minutes. Patients were given a free choice as to whether they saw the doctor or the nurse practitioner, and one of the purposes of the project was to discover whether patients presented different problems to the nurse. Research on the project indicated that most patients saw the nurse for prophylactic procedures and with general symptoms and ill-defined conditions (Stilwell 1987 and 1988). The majority of the problems presented to the nurse practitioner (60 per cent) concerned social or emotional problems, or health education. Few of the patients received a prescription from the nurse and when they were asked why they chose to see the nurse, most patients replied that it was the time and the ability of the nurse to listen to problems and provide more extensive explanations on health matters. An analysis of the public's attitudes to nurse practitioner care in this study showed that most people who had consulted the nurse practitioner would do so again. Clearly, the model of the nurse practitioner in the community is of a nurse not working to the illness or 'medical' model, but a holistic approach based on the concept of health and prevention.

The idea of a nurse with greater authority to make clinical judgements in areas of patient care previously controlled by doctors is now also spreading to hospitals. At Oldchurch Hospital in Romford experienced nurses are employed as nurse practitioners in the Accident and Emergency department (Head 1988). These nurses assess patients on arrival to the department, and have authority to refer patients who attend with inappropriate problems to other agencies such as the general practitioner. The nurse practitioners treat minor injuries them- selves and can send patients with suspected fractures direct to X-ray. The benefits to patients of this extended role for the nurses have included an enormous drop in waiting time in the department (from 10 per cent of new patients being in the department for less than an hour in 1985 to 85 per cent in 1988). Also, most patients expressed satisfaction at being initially assessed by a nurse and with the treatment they received from the nurse practitioner.

The change to nurse practitioners seems to offer a service from which patients benefit directly, and many nurses see the nurse practitioner movement as a way of advancing the occupation of nursing. However, as a result of her research and experience Stilwell concludes that 'if the role of nurse practitioner is to be developed in the British health care system, as has been advocated, then certain issues need clarification including . . . the difference between what nurse practitioners do now and what they could do, the style of nursing care that is most helpful to patients, the attitudes of doctors to professional autonomy for nurses, and the attitudes of nurses to role expansion for themselves' (Stilwell 1989). To this end Stilwell has conducted further research with nurses and patients from eight general practices. Preliminary results have helped to define a clearer role for nurse practitioners and have indicated the kind of educational preparation that nurse practitioners could benefit from (Stilwell 1989).

Lecturer practitioners

There has been a growing concern over the past decade about the disparity between what is taught in theory and what is practised in reality in nursing, sometimes called the theory–practice gap. A significant amount of research has been undertaken in this area, particularly in terms of clinical learning environments and in relation to the difficulties experienced in the use of research-based knowledge in practice. Recently, attempts have been made to explore different ways of closing this gap, partly through the introduction of a variety of new unified roles, that is, roles where the authority and responsibility for all aspects of professional practice are vested in one person. One such role is that of the lecturer practitioner.

Vaughan (1990) describes lecturer practitioners as having responsibility and authority for both practice and education with the following two aims:

(a) to identify and maintain the standards of practice and policies within a defined clincial area; and
(b) to prepare and contribute to the educational programme of students in relation to the theory and practice of nursing in that unit.

FitzGerald, herself occupying a lecturer practitioner post, describes it as: 'a senior nurse who has a mastery of practice, education, management and research. Through demonstrating these collective skills, he/she is able to lead a team delivering a professional service to patients and create the opportunities for sound learning.' (FitzGerald 1989).

Lecturer practitioner jobs are still relatively new, and as yet little research or evaluation has been completed as to their effectiveness. However, an action research study has been undertaken showing some of the strategies that are useful when establishing the role and in the preparation of the clinical area in which the job is situated (FitzGerald 1989), and a research project is underway which is examining the implementation and development of lecturer prac-titioner roles in nursing (Lathlean 1991). Findings from both these studies reinforce the importance of the lecturer practitioner in ensuring that her staff nurses have opportunities for their own professional development and are adequately prepared and supported to work with student nurses, since the viability and success of the job seems to be dependent on staff nurses being able to play a major part in the education of students as well as being autonomous practitioners in their own right. The whole subject of innovative approaches to combining theory and practice by the development of new roles is the subject of a book (Lathlean and Vaughan, forthcoming).

Keeping up with developments in nursing

Keeping abreast of new ideas and developments is the responsibility of every nurse. One way of doing so is through subscribing to a journal. It has been shown that most nurses in practice do not read journals regularly (Myco 1980), yet these can offer the most up-to-date information on nursing matters. The weekly nursing magazines tend to contain more topical news items, but also provide theoretical, pragmatic and research-based articles on all aspects of nursing. They are particularly useful for the promotion of new ideas and the description of actual experiences which may well be of use to many nurses. 'Change generators' or the leaders in nursing have the opportunity to express their views and opinions, and the time between acceptance of an article and it's publication is usually fairly short, thus ensuring the currency of the subject.

The monthly and quarterly nursing journals tend to have more in-depth articles, though some, such as *Professional Nurse* and *Senior Nurse*, have a mixture of news and articles. Other are specific to one branch of nursing – such as care of the elderly, surgical nursing or midwifery. The more 'academic' nursing journals, for example *The Journal of Advanced Nursing, The International Journal of Nursing Studies* and *Nurse Education Today* contain detailed research reports and theoretical articles and are published quarterly or bimonthly. These are expensive and thus are usually best consulted through a library. These journals, as well as many of the others, have a system for 'refereeing' articles, that is, before an article is accepted for publication it is read by at least one other person who is deemed to be knowledgeable about the subject matter. This helps to ensure the quality and accuracy of articles. However, the referee and the publisher can only make their judgements based on the sometimes fairly limited information provided, and, in the case of research-based articles, acceptance for publication is no guarantee that the research was necessarily good research. Thus whilst it is important for the writer of such articles to give sufficient detail of his methodology, the reader will need to consider them critically.

Reasons sometimes given for not reading journals are: lack of time; poor availability of certain journals; lack of knowledge of which journals are the most appropriate; inability to understand the presentation of information, especially in the more academic journals; and inability to critique articles. One way of overcoming many of these problems is for a ward to subscribe to one or more journals and for all members to be encouraged to read and share the information. A journal club, in which each member subscribes or has access to a different journal and passes it around to the others, or agrees to report back on specific articles with a view to informing others, is an effective way of covering a large number of journals.

Another way in which nurses can keep up-to-date is through attending conferences and study days. These may be held by health authorities, professional organisations, publishers and, increasingly, by private organisations. Many health authorities will allow a nurse time to attend a conference if she pays her own expenses, or will pay for the fee if she attends in her own time. These are useful, not only in relation to the formal sessions, but also for the opportunity to meet other nurses who are working in a similar area, to share information and experiences. In addition, the ward, unit or institution in which the nurse works may have a working group to consider some aspect of change, such as the implementation of primary nursing, or the promotion of quality assurance through, for example, a quality circle (see Chapter 3). As well as the nurse being able to provide a valuable contribution, this is often a good opportunity for having access to the thinking and plans of others.

Conclusion

New developments in nursing are occurring all the time. Looking to the future, more emphasis is likely to be placed on quality assurance, as referred to in Chapter 2. For example, the Dynamic Standard Setting System (Kitson *et al.* 1990), promoted by the RCN, will probably be widely implemented in the United Kingdom. This system helps clinical nurses identify and solve problems in their nursing care in an attempt to raise standards of practice. Another development could be the spreading of nursing controlled beds in hospitals. Already piloted in a few areas (see, for example, Rogers 1985 and Pearson 1988), the idea of being able to admit patients with nursing needs to beds where care is co-ordinated by other nurses is an appealing one, especially if the outcomes of that care are positive and the project is cost-effective (Pearson *et al.* 1988).

Undoubtedly, as time goes on nursing will come under even more external pressures, such as the desire for nurses to become more involved in the technology of modern medicine, and the greater push towards effectiveness and efficiency. As a result nurses will have to decide where their priorities lie. Not all change, however, is necessarily beneficial; for example, the increasing fear of litigation is already stifling nurses' autonomy and could lead to dilemmas. Such difficulties can only be resolved by both considering the patient's own views, and keeping the interests of the patient paramount.

If nursing is to move forward, then it is up to all nurses to be involved in change and to support it in their own areas. The nurses qualifying today must not become the diehards of the future. Stability and the familiar may be 'safe' whereas change and the new can produce feelings of insecurity. In the past nurses who questioned were often labelled as troublemakers, while those with ideas were described as unrealistic. However, if a constant strive for improvement in patient care is the norm, and certainly the current reforms in nurse education are encouraging the student nurse to be analytical and critical then trying out different ways of doing things and evaluating the results will become an automatic part of nursing practice.

References

Chalmers, J. (1990) 'Making resource management work', *The Professional Nurse* Vol. 5, No. 4, pp. 178–80.
Department of Health and Social Security (1986) *Neighbourhood Nursing: a Focus for Care*, Report of the Community Nursing Review, London: HMSO.

Department of Health (1989a) *Working for Patients*, London: HMSO.

Department of Health (1989b) *Caring for People*, London: HMSO.

Ersser, S. and Tutton, E. (1991) *Primary Nursing in Perspective*, London: Scutari Press.

FitzGerald, M. (1989) *Lecturer Practitioner: Action Researcher*, Unpublished Master of Nursing Thesis, University of Cardiff.

Head, S. (1988) 'Nurse practitioners: the new pioneers', *Nursing Times*, Vol. 84, No. 26, pp. 26–8.

Heineken, J. and Nussbaumer, B. (1976) 'Survival for nurses initiating change', *Supervisor Nurse*, October, pp. 52–3, 56–7.

Hersey, P. and Blanchard, K. H. (1977) *Management of Organizational Behaviour: Utilising Human Resources*. New Jersey: Prentice Hall.

Kitson, A., Hyndman, S., Harvey, G. and Yerrell, P. (1990) *Quality Patient Care: the Dynamic Standard Setting System*, London: Scutari Press.

Lathlean, J. (1989) *Policy Making in Nurse Education*, Oxford: Ashdale Press.

Lathlean, J. (1991) *The Implementation and Development of Lecturer Practitioner Roles in Nursing: Ethnography One*, Unpublished Research Report, University of Oxford, Department of Educational Studies.

Lippitt, G. L. (1973) *Visualizing Change: Model Building and the Change Process*, California: University Associates Inc.

Mauksch, I. G. and Miller, M. H. (1981) *Implementing Change in Nursing*, London: C. V. Mosby.

McMahon, R. (1990) 'Power and collegial relations among nurses on wards adopting primary nursing and hierarchical ward management structures', *Journal of Advanced Nursing*, Vol. 15, pp. 232–9.

Millar, B. (1989) 'Making sense of resource management', *Nursing Times*, Vol. 85, No. 11, pp. 26–8.

Miller, A. (1988) 'Nurse–patient dependency: is it iatrogenic?' *Journal of Advanced Nursing*, Vol. 10, No. 1, pp. 133–44.

Myco, F. (1980) 'Nursing research information: are nurses educators and practitioners seeking it out?' *Journal of Advanced Nursing*, Vol. 5, No. 5, pp. 637–46.

Nursing Times (1989) 'Focus on the NHS Review', *Nursing Times*, Vol. 85, No. 6, pp. 16–19.

Ottoway, R. N. (1982) 'Defining the change agent' in Evans, B., Powell, J. A. and Talbot, R. *Changing Design*, London: John Wiley.

Pearson, A. (ed.) (1988) *Primary Nursing: Nursing at the Burford and Oxford Nursing Development Units*, London: Croom Helm.

Pearson, A., Durand, I. and Punton, S. (1988) *Therapeutic Nursing: an Evaluation of an Experimental Nursing Unit in the British National Health Service*, Oxfordshire Health Authority.

Rogers, R. (1985) 'Nurses control care in new unit', *Senior Nurse*, Vol. 3, No. 5, p. 3.

Royal College of Nursing (1986) *Comments on the UKCC's Project 2000 proposals*, London: RCN.

Silver, H. K., Ford, L. C., Ripley, S. S. and Isoe, J. (1985) 'Perspectives twenty years after. From the pioneers of the nurse practitioner movement', *Nurse Practitioner*, Vol. 10, No. 1, pp. 15–18.

Stilwell, B. (1987) 'Different expectations', *Nursing Times*, Vol. 83, No. 24, pp. 59–61.

Stilwell, B. (1988) 'Patients' attitudes to the availability of a nurse practitioner to general practice', in Bowling, A. and Stilwell, B., *The Nurse in Family Practice*, London: Scutari Press.

Stilwell, B. (1989) 'Defining a role for nurse practitioners in British general practice', in Wilson-Barnett, J. and Robinson, S., *Directions in Nursing Research*, London: Scutari Press.

Tutton, S. and Ersser, S. (1991) 'Primary nursing: implications for the patient', in Ersser, S. and Tutton, E. (eds.) *Primary Nursing in Perspective*, London: Scutari Press.

United Kingdom Central Council for Nursing, Midwifery and Health Visiting (1986) *Project 2000: A New Preparation for Practice*, London: UKCC.

United Kingdom Central Council for Nursing, Midwifery and Health Visiting (1987) *Project 2000: The Final Proposals. Project Paper 9*, London: UKCC.

United Kingdom Central Council for Nursing, Midwifery and Health Visiting (1990) *The Report of the Post-registration Education and Practice Project*, London: UKCC.

Vaughan, B. (1990) 'Knowing what and knowing how: the role of the lecturer practitioner', in Salvage, J. and Kershaw, B. (eds.), *Models for Nursing 2*, London: Scutari Press.

Vousden, M. (1989) 'Resource management: Freeman's choice', *Nursing Times*, Vol. 85, No. 11, pp. 28–30.

Wood, K. (1990) 'Resource management in action on the ward', *The Professional Nurse*, Vol. 5, No. 5, pp. 254–8.

Further reading

Lancaster, J. and Lancaster, W. (1982) *Concepts for Advanced Nursing Practice: The Nurse as a Change Agent*, St. Louis: C. V. Mosby.

Mauksch, I. G. and Miller, M. H. (1981) *Implementing Change in Nursing*, London: C. V. Mosby.

Pearson, A. (1985) 'Nurses as change agents and a strategy for change', *Nursing Practice*, Vol. 1, No. 2, pp. 80–4.

Pearson, A. and Vaughan, B. (1984) 'Introducing change into nursing practice in the Open University Centre for Continuing Education', *A Systematic Approach to Nursing Care*, Milton Keynes: Open University Press.

Wright, S. (1989) *Changing Nursing Practice*, London: Edward Arnold.

9 Professional Development and Continuing Education

JUDITH LATHLEAN

Introduction

Newly qualified nurses are often so relieved to have completed their training, and to have passed their examinations, that the last thing on their minds is further education and training. If, at this stage, they are still committed to staying in nursing they are, in the main, keen to 'get on with the job of being a trained nurse'. Yet many feel inadequately prepared for their first staff nurse post (Lathlean *et al.* 1986; Rogers and Lawrence 1987). In addition, attitudes held, experiences gained and decisions made in the first few months of post-registration can significantly influence the career and future directions taken by the individual. For these and other reasons, a number of health authorities are providing opportunities for the consolidation of learning already achieved, and for the promotion of new skills and knowledge, through professional development schemes for staff nurses.

While special programmes aimed at newly registered nurses are still relatively new, having been pioneered mainly in the mid- to late-1980s, the importance of further education for all nurses after registration is becoming more widely recognised. 'Continuing education' tends to be the generic term used to encompass all forms of education that occur after the initial training for a profession such as nursing or teaching. Traditionally, in nursing, a broad division has been made in continuing education between post-basic and in-service education, the former being defined as those courses 'for which a nationally recognised certificate is awarded. Such courses may be in clinical nursing, teaching or management' (Rogers and Lawrence 1987). In-service education has been provided and controlled by an employing authority and does not usually involve a nationally recognised certificate, though this may be changing, for example with the linking of some courses to the National Health Service Training Authority (NHSTA) and CNAA.

This view of continuing education seems very narrow, implying attendance at formal courses. Continuing education should include a wide range of activities and opportunities, some leading to a national certificate (for example, as awarded by the English National Board or an educational institution) or a further statutory qualification (such as RMN, RNMH or RSCN), and some more oriented towards professional and personal development, including training in specific skills and the enhancement of knowledge as well as studying for a higher education degree or diploma. It should also include activities which are in fact part of everyday life such as reading professional journals, contributing to local discussion groups or searching for further information about a matter of local interest, possibly through small-scale research.

Once qualified, a large number of alternatives and choices exist in the pursuit of a career in nursing. However, some nurses on registration have no clear sense of direction, or, alternatively, have such fixed ideas about their next steps in nursing that they are unable to stand back and review how appropriate these are in the light of experience (Lathlean *et al.* 1986). Career planning is an important part of being a staff nurse and one that is obviously closely linked with decisions about, and opportunities in continuing education.

The need for further education and development

Initial nurse education is the foundation stone of a professional career, but it is only a basic introduction to the practice of nursing and just the beginning of life-long learning. It is important for the recently qualified nurse to continue to learn and develop – additional knowledge is required for the job of staff nurse, as well as the opportunity to examine current practices critically and to keep abreast of new information and ideas.

The UKCC Code of Conduct (UKCC 1984) states that every nurse, in exercising professional accountability, should:

> take every reasonable opportunity to maintain and improve professional knowledge and competence [and] acknowledge any limitations of competence and refuse in such cases to accept delegated functions without first having received instruction in regard to those functions and having been assessed as competent.

The Council further adds, in the report of the Post-registration Education and Practice Project – PREPP (UKCC 1990b), that 'all nurses, midwives and health visitors must demonstrate that they have maintained and developed their professional knowledge and competence'.

This recommendation is not new in its sentiment since the debate about updating knowledge and skills has been going on for some time. A report from the National Staff Committee (1981) stated that:

> Every individual nurse of whatever grade or sphere of work should be aware of the need to update and expand her knowledge and skills. Fundamental in this is the need to assess critically her own learning needs, search and find appropriate resources and become self-directing in respect of her own learning.

In the past many registered nurses have given little time to continuing education; the majority have undertaken no formal courses since they qualified and, for various reasons, many nurses do not even read the journals regularly. Whilst PREPP and other sources are now placing an increasing emphasis on the responsibility of the individual in her own continuing education, educational institutions and employing authorities must share this responsibility by providing appropriate courses and other learning opportunities and the chance for staff to participate in them. A survey conducted in 1988 of a representative sample of district health authorities showed that only 38 per cent of districts had a philosophy for continuing professional education, and a similar percentage had a policy (Rogers et al. 1989). Furthermore, the provision made by health authorities in continuing education varies greatly, reflecting different attitudes towards its importance as well as a wide disparity in resources. A national survey of continuing professional education indicated that, in the 175 health districts responding, the number of staff involved in delivering in-service and post-basic education ranged from one to more than fifteen, less than half ran in-service management and teaching courses regularly, and only 2 per cent ran health education courses (Rogers and Lawrence 1987).

The statutory and professional bodies in nursing are keen to promote the importance of continuing education for the registered nurse. The aim of the United Kingdom Central Council is to complement the reformed initial nursing education – Project 2000 – by a new 'coherent and comprehensive framework incorporating the standards and principles of education and practice beyond registration to meet the needs of patients, clients and health service' (UKCC 1989), and to this end it set up the Post-registration Education and Practice Project – PREPP. A paper was prepared (UKCC 1990a) and, following a period of discussion with the profession and others, a report was issued (UKCC 1990b). This report raises a number of very important notions for nursing which are intended as statutory requirements including the following:

- the need for nurses to demonstrate the maintenance and development of their professional knowledge and competence;
- the need for individuals to record professional development in a personal profile;
- the requirement that all practitioners complete a period of study or provide evidence of appropriate learning during the three years leading to periodic registration, with a minimum of five days' study leave being undertaken every three years;
- the necessity for all nurses with a break of five years or more who wish to return to complete a return to practice programme.

Alongside the work of the UKCC in producing professional standards for education and practice, the English National Board has agreed to produce a framework for continuing professional education in nursing, midwifery and health visiting which is informed by research. There are three parts to this initiative, planned to take place between 1989 and 1992: a needs assessment study and the development of a framework for continuing education; the development of a system for accreditation; and a consideration of the greater use of open learning. This work, together with PREPP, signifies a major change in attitudes towards continuing education and is likely to have considerable impact on the profession's expectations of registered nurses.

Opportunities for development

As already indicated, continuing education is not just about attendance at courses and formal events. It also includes a wide range of activities – formal and informal – which lead to increased knowledge and professional and personal growth. Fig. 9.1 illustrates some of the different opportunities for learning.

Obviously, different activities are suitable for meeting different needs. The identification of what is required should come from the individual in the first instance, and whilst the individual can take much of the initiative for action, successful outcomes are dependent on a shared approach and a number of different contributory factors. Rogers and Lawrence (1987) identified four factors as important in the development of skills and interests within a post: the post itself (does it provide scope, is it challenging?); the attitudes of managers (do they encourage the individual to develop their skills, to make the most of opportunities for learning?); personal motivation (do I feel keen to pursue my professional interests, am I prepared/able to invest time, energy and money in my professional and personal growth?); and finance/resources (is time and money available to pursue opportunities, is staffing sufficient to allow time out for continuing education?). All these factors are interlinked, however. For example, if managers – wards sisters and senior nurse managers – have a positive and flexible attitude to continuing education, with an understanding that it is essential for motivating individuals and in some cases preventing burnout, they will ensure that opportunities are created even when resources are limited and staffing low.

Further research by Rogers et al. (1989) highlighted the need for a partnership at all stages in the organisation and provision of continuing professional education between the qualified nurse, her service-based colleagues and education staff. Most of the informal and 'in-service' opportunities can be agreed between the individual and her immediate manager, usually the ward sister. However, if study leave and/or funding is required, the request needs to be negotiated through, and agreed with, the nursing officer or senior nurse manager. In this respect, some nurses feel that all

Fig. 9.1   Potential opportunities for learning and continuing education
(Adapted from Dodwell and Lathlean 1989)

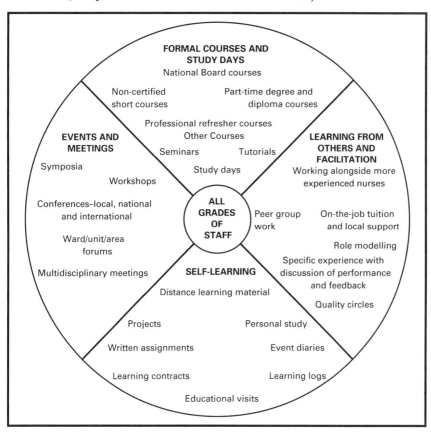

continuing education should be conducted in 'work' time and with the
employer's resources. Conversely, others are prepared to give up their own
time and to provide some or all of the necessary resources. The *shared*
responsibility for professional development and continuing education suggests
that a balance needs to be struck between these two points.

Professional development schemes for newly qualified nurses

One of the most significant changes affecting the opportunities for development
of the newly qualified nurse has been the establishment of special professional
development programmes aimed at this group of nurses. Many such schemes
stemmed from, or were encouraged by, an initiative taken by the Department
of Health in 1981, when, as an outcome of a seminar in Harrogate, attended by
nurses from many aspects of nursing, it was recommended that:

a newly registered nurse should have a period of professional consolidation and development following registration. This period would consist of supervised and supported practice in a designated training area and would take the form of a 'core professional module' – applicable to nurses in any branch of nursing.

(DHSS 1982).

Three of the resulting schemes were evaluated (Lathlean *et al.* 1986) and the progress in a number of others was discussed regularly in a national forum. The research showed the main requirements to be as follows:

- the involvement of nurses in identifying their own needs, and in planning to meet those needs;
- the regular review of progress between the individual, the manager and/or others such as a tutor;
- an emphasis on ward/practice-based learning related to the nurse's actual role;
- the opportunity for group membership with peers, preferably with a facilitator, to share skills, knowledge and experience;
- the provision of support and guidance from outside the ward;
- some time away from the ward for discussion and reflection.

Whilst a number of health authorities do already provide formal input through study days and seminars, either especially for their newly qualified nurses or for trained nurses with a range of experience, most of these features can be achieved without formal courses as such. Nevertheless, planning and the provision of some resources, such as the time away from practice, are necessary.

A useful part of this more systematic approach to professional development is the individualised plan of action for gaining the relevant experience, knowledge and skills. Such a plan, usually developed and agreed jointly between an individual and a more senior, experienced nurse (sometimes referred to as a mentor) – or a tutor – can comprise a range of different learning opportunities. (This is a similar process to the one recommended by UKCC in PREPP – the adoption of personal profiles for all registered nurses.) Fig. 9.2 shows a typical plan for a nurse's first year after qualification.

The whole area of professional development is relatively new and changing rapidly. For example, many health authorities are now developing a 'core' professional development programme, to prevent overlap between different specialties, including issues such as research, changing work organisation, ethics, and so on. Furthermore, UKCC are now recommending 'a period of support for all newly registered practitioners to consolidate the competencies or learning outcomes achieved at registration' and the provision of a preceptor to give support to each newly registered practitioner (UKCC 1990b). Therefore, it is important for the newly registered nurse to explore the options available to

Fig. 9.2   Professional development plan for Nurse Smith

Participation in courses/study days, etc.
● Six professional development seminars for newly qualified nurses (role of the staff nurse, accountability, managing nursing work, teaching and learning, legal and ethical issues, research in practice).
● Primary nursing module (organised by the school of nursing).

Attendance at conferences/seminars
● Locally based annual research conference: 'Research into Practice'.
● Seminar on 'Symptom Control for Dying Patients' run by local hospice.

Role modelling and related activities
● Work with Senior Staff Nurse Brown to observe and learn about nursing care of patient receiving total parenteral nutrition.
● Observe Staff Nurse Green planning discharge of patient.
● Plan off-duty rota with Senior Staff Nurse Brown.
● Follow discharged patient into the community and work with relevant District Nurse for a day.

Extended role
● Intravenous drug administration assessment (following professional development seminars, according to the hospital policy).

Self-directed activities and learning
● Self-reflective diary keeping note of critical incidents for first three months of job (to be discussed with Senior Staff Nurse Brown (mentor) or Sister White when feedback is required).
● Read *The Professional Nurse* monthly and skim *Nursing Times* for relevant articles weekly.
● Work through the Open University package, P553 – *A Systematic Approach to Nursing Care* and take part in Group Sessions with peers from the professional development programme.

Future plans
● Apply for ENB Course 998, *Teaching and Assessing in Clinical Practice*.
● Attend two-day workshop on 'Preparation for Mentoring', run by the school, and work through training package, if chosen to be a mentor for the new Project 2000 students.

---

her because they vary greatly from place to place and new schemes are being started all the time. As well as consulting local sources (such as the school or nursing or local colleges), information can also be sought from the English National Board Careers Service in Sheffield* or from the other National Boards.

Specialist clinical courses

Following the initial period as a staff nurse – and a requirement for entry into a number of the courses is a minimum of six-months' post-registration experience – some nurses consider undertaking a specialist clinical nursing course. These are approved by the National Boards and are designed to help people understand the specialty of their choice. At present there are two types of course: 'long' certificated courses which help to prepare for work in a particular area of nursing – with formal assessment – and 'short' statement of attendance courses (up to thirty days and normally part-time) to keep nurses up-to-date with current trends or deepen understanding of a specific area of care – usually without formal assessment.

Unfortunately, these courses are oversubscribed and many are heavily booked in advance. Therefore, careful thought in the choice of which to apply for is prudent and the preparedness to wait for acceptance.

Further qualifications

A first-level registered nurse can train for other parts of the Register in a shorter time than is required for a new entrant – typically from one year to eighteen months. However, with the advent of Project 2000, the requirements for nurses trained under the old system who wish to gain a further qualification have been reviewed. Nurses in that position are advised to obtain up-to-date information on the new regulations.

Midwifery training is a popular choice of many nurses, often because it is believed to be the pathway to a number of different specialties in nursing, and it is needed if the nurse wishes to practise in certain other countries. However, it can be more appropriate for individuals to undertake one of the above-mentioned specialist clinical courses in preference. At present, only first-level RGN nurses can gain access to the shortened eighteen-months training; others are required to undertake the full three-year training.

Nursing in the community offers a range of different opportunities including district nursing, community psychiatric nursing, community nursing for people with mental handicaps, health visiting, school nursing, practice nursing, health education and occupational health. Different courses are available for all these

* Information can be obtained from: ENB Careers, PO Box 356, Sheffield, S8 0SJ.

specialisms and whilst a qualification is not an essential requirement for some (e.g. to work as a practice nurse or in health education), the relevant training is desirable, as is a certain type of experience gained prior to undertaking the qualification and seeking to practise.

Higher education

The opportunities for nurses to participate in higher education and to gain a formal academic qualification which is recognised both within and outside nursing are steadily increasing. This whole area is under considerable focus at present and the next few years are likely to see great change. For example, registered nurses have been able to undertake the Diploma in Nursing, validated by the Universities of London/Wales as a part-time three-year course organised in six units over three years, but, since 1986, a two-year programme has been phased in and this will eventually replace the three-year course (for discussions of one of the pilot schemes for the two-year Diploma, see Smyth 1988 and McSweeney 1989). In addition, the Diploma of Nursing can be studied by open learning (for example, through the Distance Learning Centre, Polytechnic of the South Bank). Alternatively it is possible to opt for the Diploma in Professional Studies in Nursing (DPSN), validated by CNAA, entailing two years of part-time study. Many polytechnics (thirteen in England in 1990) are offering a four-year part-time degree in nursing, whereby either entry is restricted to holders of the DPSN or the degree course incorporates a DPSN as an intermediate award.

One of the biggest developments has been the growth of the CNAA's Credit Accumulation Transfer Scheme (CATS). This scheme was established on a pilot basis in March 1986 to give a more flexible system of higher education, and provide additional opportunities for individuals to study for degrees and diplomas. It allows students to gain credits for certain study and experience which may count towards a degree or post-graduate qualification. The CATS 'credit tariff system' divides the amount of study necessary for completion of a first degree into 360 credit points at three different levels, equivalent to the three years of a full-time degree. CNAA has been negotiating with professional organisations in relation to this scheme, and, for example, agreement has been reached with the English National Board that nurses can gain academic recognition for many of the ENB qualifications they have obtained, and credit towards the achievement of academic qualifications in nursing and related studies (CNAA 1989).

The opportunity to gain first degrees through modular schemes, or through credit accumulation, is increasingly dramatically and for those who are even more ambitious, studying for a higher degree (at Master's or Doctorate level) is a possibility. The normal requirement for entry to such programmes is possession of a first degree, but evidence of equivalent work is becoming more usual as an acceptance criterion.

Open and distance learning

In the last few years, open learning material especially written for nurses has become more available, and distance learning opportunities have increased enormously. It is usually a very cost-effective way of learning (though one where the cost often falls on the individual), and it allows study to be tailored to the individual in terms of content, time and pace. It can provide knowledge of a particular kind, or lead to a qualification such as a diploma or degree, but it is often most effective when combined with a method of interactive learning, such as group discussions, or working with a facilitator or tutor for part of the time.

Perhaps the organisation best known for promoting distance learning is the Open University (OU). For some time, the OU has had a battery of courses and study packs that either form part of its undergraduate programme, its associate student programme, or can be purchased and followed by anyone interested in the subject. They include such topics as reducing the risk of coronary heart disease or cancer, and drug use and misuse as well as many in health-related areas such as disability, ageing, children and the family. They also have plans for a new Diploma in Health and Social Welfare which will be an undergraduate-level diploma of two credit equivalents. Students on this programme must study three core courses and complete a project (together attracting one full credit), but there will be considerable flexibility over the other courses that can be pursued to gain the second full credit. This new Diploma, which will be available from 1992 onwards, is very much planned with credit transfer in mind.

The Open University by no means has the monopoly on open learning. Another scheme called Delivering Health Care (formerly Health PICKUP) is jointly funded by the National Health Service Training Authority and the Department of Education and Science. This is a flexible, modular programme of non-clinical post-basic training, based on principles of open learning, for qualified members of the nursing profession and professions allied to medicine across England and Wales. It is skills-based and derived from extensive research across the service. The initial modules include the following:

● The role of the professional in charge.
● Setting objectives and standards for care.
● Assessing needs and priorities.
● Managing the caseload and time.
● Helping staff learn through experience.
● Working with other professionals.

In addition, the National Health Service Training Authority is piloting a new degree in health studies in conjunction with CNAA. Such a degree, which uses open learning methods, is likely to be available from 1995.

Open and distance learning is a major area of growth. As a particular learning style it does not suit everyone, though its increasing availability has created a great many opportunities for a much larger number of people (Rogers *et al.* 1989). The subject is covered comprehensively and usefully by Robinson (1989).

Career planning and options

For the new nurse, just taking up a staff nurse post, the range of possibilities in nursing may seem overwhelming. Lathlean *et al.*'s (1986) study suggested that newly registered nurses need:

> information about opportunities open to them; help to explore common assumptions about suitable career paths and assistance in viewing the context of their work more broadly. Second they require individual guidance in thinking through their own plans, especially from someone who knows them sufficiently well to give them accurate feedback about their capabilities, . . . and guidance and support in putting their plans into action.

Other research has shown that surprisingly little career guidance is available to registered nurses (Schober 1988). Schober's study indicated that career guidance needs to be related to a system of performance appraisal, yet 80 per cent of her respondents, who were attending Royal College of Nursing courses, had not had a performance appraisal since registration (Schober 1987). In the scheme studied by Lathlean, support came jointly from the tutors and the sisters who were involved in the scheme. Informal help also came out of group discussions with peers. Although the most appropriate person to help a nurse make decisions about her career is usually the immediate manager, sometimes it is easier for an individual to be more open about her aspirations with someone to whom she is not accountable (such as a tutor or a personnel nurse). Further, Bracken and Davis (1989) suggest that a 'mentor' can be helpful to an individual in helping her to plan a career. Indeed, they argue that in the United States, people who have been mentored reach senior positions much faster, up to two years ahead of those who have not (Gallaher cited in Bracken and Davis, 1989). This is of course assuming that the mentor is in a position to assist the 'mentee' to identify her strengths and weaknesses and to clarify her preferences, and is knowledgeable about possible options.

Information about career opportunities is often available through the school of nursing, or the health authority library. Alternatively, the ENB has a careers advisory service. Other sources of information include careers 'conventions' held occasionally by national nursing journals and the like.

Clinical practice

Traditionally, in nursing, 'moving up' and 'promotion' has been associated with moving further away from clinical practice into aspects such as management, teaching or even research. One of the intentions of the implementation of a new structure for clinical grades has been to encourage nurses to stay in clinical practice, and reward them accordingly. Although there are many anomalies in the clinical grading structures it is possible for junior nurses to work towards highly graded, but clinically based, posts.

Further, there is an increasing recognition of the importance and centrality of clinical practice whereby high-level clinical nursing skills and knowledge are valued, rather than thought of as 'inferior' to teaching or management skills. Hence the establishment of well-graded clinical specialist posts and suggestions that there should be senior clinical practitioners (RCN 1983; DHSS 1988; UKCC 1990a). A parallel – though different – development is that of posts that combine advanced nursing expertise, and educational and management knowledge and skills, often referred to as 'lecturer practitioners'. A lecturer practitioner is a person who:

> manages a clinical unit, sets the policies and styles of work organisation, develops the staff and has authority for such things as skill mix within the budget. She is a clinical expert who acts as a consultant for the other practitioners while maintaining her own practice in a variety of ways. She also has responsibility for teaching both the theory and practice of nursing within the clinical setting.
>
> (Vaughan 1989)

Ideally, the lecturer practitioner should be someone with considerable clinical experience, since this is the core of the role, as well as managerial expertise and a teaching qualification. Whilst the change to such roles has not been easy, it is clearly an important and challenging trend in nursing. Lecturer practitioners are discussed further in Chapter 9.

Teaching

To pursue a career as nurse teacher, proper planning is required as there are a number of stages to go through. These are outlined in an article by Buttigieg (1990). Currently, to be able to record a teaching qualification with UKCC, the nurse must have a minimum of three years' full-time clinical experience (or equivalent part-time) in the ten years before recording a qualification on the register, at least two years of which should have been in a post of responsibility and in an area where initial or post-registration students are allocated regularly. This latter requirement is considered to be especially important.

In addition, a potential candidate must provide evidence of further professional knowledge beyond initial training, normally through completion of an approved course lasting no less than six months. This means that the prospective nurse teacher is likely to take an ENB course in teaching and assessing in clinical practice (or similar, but, according to Buttigieg (1990), the City and Guilds Course 730 is not an acceptable prerequisite for teacher training except for some clinical teachers) followed by the Diploma in Nursing or the Diploma in Professional Studies in Nursing, or possibly a part-time modular degree course, with a full-time final year to enable participants to get a teaching qualification as well. The ENB now approves seven teacher training courses at first degree level.

Each of the National Boards not only sets its own criteria for entry to teacher training but approves its own courses. In England the Board approves over twenty courses but an attempt is being made to gain a more equitable geographical spread (Buttigieg 1990). All these are validated by CNAA or a university. They fall into a number of types: full-time including Certificate in Education (FE), Post-Graduate Certificate in Education of Adults and a BEd (Honours) Degree in Nursing Education, part-time Certificates in Education and mixed mode full- and part-time modular degree courses in Nursing with Education or Nursing Education. New courses are being approved; up-to-date information on these courses can be gained from the relevant National Boards.

In addition, it is possible to train as a midwife teacher, a district nurse tutor (practical work teacher), or a health visitor tutor (fieldwork teacher), all of which need the relevant professional qualification as a prerequisite for training. An insight into practical work teacher and fieldwork teacher training can be gained from a research study which evaluated their education and preparation (Maggs and Purr 1989).

Management

It has been argued that management and managing form a part of the role of all qualified nurses (see Chapter 3) and thus development of management skills is necessary for all grades of nurse. However, some nurses will choose to work eventually in formally designated management posts and whilst there is no prescribed route or qualification a number of alternatives are of benefit. Nearly all health authorities have established 'management training' programmes, some aspects of which are 'in-house'; others are provided by local colleges and a variety of institutions.

Normally, three 'levels' of management training are offered: foundation courses; middle management courses; and senior management courses. Foundation management courses may well be appropriate for staff nurses, whereas middle and senior management are normally oriented to sister grade and above. In addition, preparation for general management posts is provided by the NHSTA General Management Training Schemes (GMTS).

There are other avenues, too, that are not specific to nursing. For example, it is possible to study for a Diploma in Management Studies or Personnel Management or even a degree in business studies. The advantage of such generic courses is the applicability of the knowledge on a much wider basis than nursing, though their often inevitable orientation towards business and commerce may prove to be a challenge. There is, however, an increasing number of professionals from the various public sector organisations undertaking such courses, and the opportunity to discuss issues in multidisciplinary and multiprofessional groups is valuable.

Research

It is artificial to separate out research from practice and teaching, in that nurses nowadays are constantly being urged to use research thinking to critique and challenge current practice and research knowledge as a basis for their teaching (MacGuire 1990). However, the opportunities to undertake actual research at some time in a career, or to be involved in a small project which entails using or testing out research findings, have increased greatly in recent years. For many, they arise as part of a degree or diploma course. Sometimes this stimulates a deep interest in research, and for those keen to specialise in it there are a few designated research posts within health authorities at hospital, district and regional level. Also, there are a number of nursing departments and research units employing nurses to undertake, or participate in, research projects. Sometimes, limited research experience only is required since the post has a training element. Increasingly, though, nurses specialising in research will have at least a first degree and often a higher degree.

As research knowledge and methods become embedded in both initial preparation and continuing education, research awareness will become an important facet of the role of all nurses, in that nurses will be expected to use research to develop their practice. In many instances they may also be expected to be involved in or even to undertake research as part of their remit or job description, as has been the case in medicine for many years. There is an increasing emphasis now on combining research with other roles, such as the researcher who is also a teacher (Wilson-Barnett 1990) and the practitioner who is also a researcher, for example FitzGerald (1989), who used action research to study and develop her lecturer practitioner role.

Conclusion

Nursing is undergoing great changes and challenges, for example as a result of the implementation of Project 2000 proposals, through the restructuring of clinical grades, by the increasing use of forms of nursing organisation such as primary nursing, and by the shifting emphasis towards self-learning and self-reflection. This has implications for the type of preparation for practice, for the actual role of the newly qualified nurse of the future, and for their development beyond registration.

In striving to achieve professional accountability and autonomy, and in the interests of offering a safe, effective and high standard service, continuous up-dating, education and development is important. The responsibility for identifying needs on a regular basis and for ensuring that these are met should be shared between the individual nurse and her employing organisation. Continuing education, in all its various forms, can also have a motivating and refreshing effect, providing new energy, differing perspectives and a vital antidote to professional and personal burnout.

References

Bracken, E. and Davis, J. (1989) 'The implications of mentorship in nursing career development', *Senior Nurse*, Vol. 9, No. 5, pp. 15–16.

Buttigieg, M. (1990) 'Learning to teach', *Nursing Times*, Vol. 86, No. 28, pp. 44–5.

Council For National Academic Awards (1989) *The Work of the Credit Accumulation and Transfer Scheme (CATS)*, London: CNAA

Department of Health and Social Security (1982) *Professional Development in Clinical Nursing – the 1980s*, London: DHSS.

Department of Health and Social Security (1988) *The Way Ahead – Career Pathways for Nurses, Midwives and Health Visitors*, London: DHSS.

Dodwell, M. and Lathlean, J. (1989) *Management and Professional Development for Nurses*, London: Harper and Row.

FitzGerald, M. (1989) *Action Researcher: Lecturer Practitioner*, Unpublished Master of Nursing Thesis, University of Cardiff.

Lathlean, J., Smith, G. and Bradley, S. (1986) *Post-Registration Development Schemes Evaluation*, Kings College, University of London.

Lathlean, J. and Vaughan, B. (eds.) (in press) *Bridging the Gap: Unifying nursing practice and theory*, London: Harper Collins.

MacGuire, J. (1990) 'Putting research findings into practice: research utilization as an aspect of the management of change', *Journal of Advanced Nursing*, Vol. 15, pp. 614–20.

Maggs, C. and Purr, B. (1989) *An Evaluation of the Education and Preparation of Fieldwork and Practical Work Teachers in England*, Oxford: Ashdale Press.

McSweeney, P. (1989) 'Three into two equals success', *Nursing Times*, Vol. 85, No. 36, pp. 74–5.

National Staff Committee for Nurses and Midwives (1981) *Recommendations on the Organisation and Provision of Continuing In-service Education and Training*, London: DHSS.

Robinson, K. (ed.) (1989) *Open and Distance Learning for Nurses*, Longman: Essex.

Rogers, J. and Lawrence, J. (1987) *Continuing Professional Education for Qualified Nurses, Midwives and Health Visitors*, Peterborough: Ashdale Press.

Rogers, J., Maggs, C. and Lawrence, J. (1989) *Distance Learning Materials for Continuing Professional Education for Qualified Nurses, Midwives and Health Visitors*, Institute of Education, University of London.

Royal College of Nursing (1983) *Towards a New Professional Structure for Nursing*, London: RCN.

Schober, J. (1987) 'Lighting the way', *Nursing Times*, Vol. 83, No. 49, pp. 66–7.

Schober, J. (1988) *The Career Guidance Experiences of Registered Nurses*, Unpublished Master of Nursing Thesis, University of Cardiff.

Smyth, T. (1988) 'Three into two will go – reshaping the diploma in nursing', *Senior Nurse*, Vol. 8, No. 9/10, pp. 22–4.

United Kingdom Central Council for Nursing, Midwifery and Health Visiting (1984) *Code of Professional Conduct for the Nurse, Midwife and Health Visitor*, London: UKCC.

United Kingdom Central Council for Nursing, Midwifery and Health Visiting (1989) *Post-Registration Education and Practice Project (PREPP)*, Circular PREPP/01, London: UKCC.

United Kingdom Central Council for Nursing, Midwifery and Health Visiting (1990a) *Discussion Paper on Post-Registration Education and Practice (January)*, London: UKCC.

United Kingdom Central Council for Nursing, Midwifery and Health Visiting (1990b) *The Report of the Post-Registration Education and Practice Project (PREPP)*, London: UKCC.

Vaughan, B. (1989) 'Two roles, one job', *Nursing Times*, Vol. 85, No. 11, p.52.

Wilson-Barnett, J. (1990) 'Integrating nursing research and practice – the role of researcher as teacher', *Journal of Advanced Nursing*, Vol. 15, pp. 621–5.

Further reading

Baker, J. (1988) *What Next: Post-Basic Opportunities for Nurses*, London: Macmillan Education.

Kershaw, B. (ed.) (1990) *Nursing Competence: A Guide to Professional Development*, London: Edward Arnold.

Lathlean, J. (1988) 'Policy issues in continuing education for clinical nurses', in White, R. (ed.) *Political Issues in Nursing: Past, Present and Future, Volume 3*, Chichester: John Wiley.

Vaughan, B. (1989) 'Career structures and staff support roles', in Vaughan, B. and Pillmoor, M. (eds.), *Managing Nursing Work*, London: Scutari Press.

Index

Page numbers in **bold** indicate primary entries